Praise for

GUT PUNCH

"A powerful recollection of a caregiver's experiences that balances advice with reflection."

—*Kirkus Reviews,* Our Verdict: "Get It"

"Pennington writes with unflinching honesty about standing beside someone you love as they fight for their life. As a family member of a cancer survivor, I know firsthand how rarely that experience is captured truthfully—and Pennington gets it exactly right. His perspective cuts through the platitudes to reveal the messy, terrifying reality of the journey itself. In sharing his darkest moments and deepest fears, he has given voice to what so many of us feel but cannot say. *Gut Punch* is a testament to love in its most tested form."

—Chris Petersen, head football coach, University of Washington/ Boise State, Fox Sports studio analyst

"Pennington has provided a moving account of the experiences of an often unacknowledged participant in cancer care—the caregiver, support person, or as he terms it, the 'sentry' for the cancer patient. He poignantly describes the trauma, despair, and ultimate redemption that he experienced when this role was thrust upon him as his wife battled an aggressive cancer and endured the harms of treatment. His story provides deep insight to aid caregivers supporting cancer patients and for medical personnel who might otherwise be only dimly aware of caregivers' struggles and needs deserving of our recognition and care."

—Dr. Donald Northfelt, MD, MS, FACP, Mayo Clinic oncology

"A moving and courageous look at the unseen strength of caregivers. Honest, compassionate, and deeply impactful. Having lived this from a survivor's point of view, this is a must read for anyone who has loved, supported, or stood strong through cancer."

—Chuck Pagano, NFL head coach, author of *Sidelined*

"Pennington's *Gut Punch* gives voice to the moment life fractures and to the long, complicated road caregivers walk afterward. With vulnerability and clarity, he reveals how love, fear, resilience, and exhaustion can coexist in the caregiving experience. He offers language for emotions that many people struggle to name. As both a mental health therapist and a CEO working at the intersection of relationships and well-being, I see firsthand how invisible the caregiver's burden can be. This memoir offers validation, perspective, and hope for anyone learning to live in a 'new normal.'"

—Kieri Olmstead, LFMT, founder and CEO of Sova Dating & Simple Empathy

"Finally, an honest account of what it costs to support a loved one battling cancer. When his beloved wife is diagnosed, Pennington wholeheartedly gives it all to care for her. Worth it, but the cost is higher than anything he expected. Reading this book, I was invited into the vulnerability of helplessness that overwhelms those of us used to being strong. The author is not the one with cancer but is convinced he has to give it all in the fight. What happens next? What happens when he too ends up paying the cost? Highly recommended for anyone who is loving someone through a life-threatening illness."

—Fr Jack Bentz, SJ and podcast host, *Catholics in Ordinary Times*

"Every great team depends on trust, sacrifice, and showing up when it truly matters. In *Gut Punch*, Paul shares a story about doing exactly that for his family. His honesty and vulnerability make this both powerful and relatable. It's a meaningful reminder that real strength isn't about control—it's about commitment to the people you love."

—Kevin Pangos, college All-American and professional basketball player

"*Gut Punch* is an emotional and heartfelt reflection encompassing a courageous journey through cancer. From diagnosis to treatment and recovery, it is written from the unique perspective of the caregiver—the guardian, the protector, the 'sentry.' Following the battle, Paul finds himself searching for identity and purpose in a new normal. *Gut Punch* offers valuable insight and perspectives for past, present, and future caregivers and provides a deeper understanding and appreciation to those who have endured this battle. Readers will be educated, entertained, and enlightened!"

—Dr. Jeffrey M. Sanwick, M.D.

"As Paul's friend, I've long admired his servant heart. But walking with someone you love through a fight for her life is a different kind of service altogether, and Paul captures it with extraordinary honesty—along with Wendi's remarkable courage. *Gut Punch* takes you through the fear, the waiting, and the miracle moment that makes you want to stand and cheer, and then into the quieter, more complicated terrain that follows survival. What moved me most is the beauty he discovers on the other side: colors more vivid, moments sharper, presence deeper. This book is a lifeline and a companion for the next sentry."

—Jared Hertz, Gonzaga Athletics

"A passionate memoir from a caregiver's perspective as he navigates through his wife's cancer diagnosis and treatments. Each chapter walks you through their 'normal' life together and the *Gut Punch* they never saw coming. More often than not, caregivers get lost in the chaos, and when the dust settles, they are ultimately left with an abundance of emotional trauma. Paul Wayne Pennington allows you inside his journey of determination, dedication, and unexpected personal growth. A must read for anyone."

—Dr. Michael Dolby, DDS and keynote speaker on personal development

"*Gut Punch* is the author's account of navigating his wife's harrowing battle against aggressive breast cancer. Paul, an inexperienced caregiver, is suddenly thrust into a role he never anticipated, becoming his wife's steadfast guardian. As he faces the challenge of supporting her through brutal chemotherapy, he tamps down his own emotions, silencing his own fears and sadness in order to be strong for his wife and those around him. The emotional weight of all he endures gradually erodes his spirit, but this too is overlooked while Paul dutifully presses on. What unfolds is a poignant exploration of love and the hidden toll of caregiving. After his wife emerges from her ordeal with a renewed zest for life, Paul finds himself in an unexpected void, struggling with feelings of numbness and isolation. He endures this for years before a wilderness trip to the Grand Canyon awakens in Paul the realization of his own deep emptiness. This leads him to finally seek help for himself.

"*Gut Punch* serves as a vital guide for male caregivers and their supporters in a society that often discourages men from expressing their emotions—especially fear, grief, or vulnerability. Paul's honest narrative sheds light on the importance of embracing and expressing our emotions without shame. This brave account not only highlights the complexity of caregiving but also champions the idea that acknowledging our emotional struggles is essential to human flourishing. Through Paul's journey, readers will find a compassionate road map for navigating love, caregiving, and emotional resilience."

—Jennifer Hassel, author of *Badass Grief: Changing Gears, Moving Forward*

"Pennington takes us on a visceral journey through the shock, prolonged stress, and lingering trauma of his wife's battle with cancer. He describes his role as that of a sentry, forever watchful, waiting to spring into action. But that tense patience comes at a cost. After the end of the harrowing treatment—this reader will never forget the 'Red Devil,' a cancer drug so powerful it left his wife sweating red droplets—Pennington opens up about his battle with depression and complete depletion. His marriage is forever changed by the experience, and even as his wife consciously strides forward, making a point not to look back, Pennington describes how difficult it was for him to claw his way back to some kind of normalcy. Cancer is difficult. So is surviving it."

—Alberto Botello, author of *180 Days* and *Spin Cycle*

"Paul Pennigton delivers his own gut punch to the reader through this powerful tale told true about love, loss, and resilience. Written in first person, this narrative is a fast-moving, emotional read. Paul's healing comes in the retelling, and we are all the more fortunate to have been invited to bear witness to these most intimate events in his life."

—Sally Dukes, author of *drummer girl*

"Singular in its blend of stoicism and deep vulnerability, Pennington alchemizes both his introspection and pain into purpose. Told in reverent and thoughtful prose, it illuminates the labyrinthine path of cancer treatment, one in which lives are changed irrevocably."

—Sarah Hughes, aspiring author and passionate reader

Gut Punch
by Paul Wayne Pennington

ISBN 979-8-89747-065-5

Edited by Miranda Dillon
Cover design by Josh Frederick

Published by

köehlerbooks™

3705 Shore Drive
Virginia Beach, VA 23455
800-435-4811
www.koehlerbooks.com

GUT PUNCH

A Caregiver's Life After Normal

PAUL WAYNE PENNINGTON

VIRGINIA BEACH
CAPE CHARLES

"Things turn out best for the people who make the best of the way things turn out."

–Coach John Wooden

NORMAL, UNTIL IT ISN'T

Normal doesn't dissolve slowly. It snaps. It slides. It shifts sideways when you aren't looking. And when you least expect it.

Sometimes it's a blink. Sometimes it's a wrong turn. And sometimes it's a phone call you wish you never answered.

Most days, normal is loyal. Predictable. Something you can count on. The silent framework that lets you walk through a day unguarded.

Until, suddenly, it isn't.

Sometimes you feel the shift coming—a tremor of intuition you brush aside. Other times it breaks open in an instant, splitting life into *before* and *after* with something as ordinary as the ringing of a phone. Or the soft slide of elevator doors.

And when it happens—when normal slips out from under you—you don't rise to meet it. You fall into it. And your new normal begins.

Elevator Down

June 29, 2021

The elevator doors slid shut, and I hit the button for the ground floor. A normal movement in a normal world. Except in our world, nothing was normal.

Wendi stood beside me, frail and unsteady. Her loose-fitting top draped over her body, chosen selectively, not with an attentive eye toward fashion but rather to keep from rubbing against the chemo port embedded in her chest. The wig—borrowed from a new friend within the Pink Ribbon Brigade—sat slightly askew, a poor disguise for the toll this battle was taking. She was pale, dizzy. I tightened my arm around her waist, steadying her uncertain legs.

Without warning, I felt pressure against my arm. A sudden, dead weight was leaning against me. I turned just in time to see her eyes roll white. Her knees buckled, and her shoulders slumped.

I caught her because, by now, I knew how to catch her. Muscle memory. Earned experience. I eased her down, letting her body strategically rest against the elevator wall. She was unconscious but breathing. That was my first calculation. My second was already running through a maze within my mind. How would I get her out of the elevator, through two sets of doors, and into the car as quickly as possible?

I had already moved the car to the front of the building, parking in the space closest to the exit door. One less obstacle ahead. Now it was keys, doors, timing. I was running through the checklist when the elevator dinged.

The doors slid open.

A young man in work boots and a tool belt stood on the other side, ready for whatever job had brought him to this elevator. His eyes first met mine, then drifted down to Wendi—bald, topless, slumped against the wall of the elevator. His mouth parted slightly, his brain scrambling to process what he was seeing.

Poor guy. Wrong elevator, wrong time.

"Hey," I said, breaking the silence and the stare. "Can you hold the doors?"

Grateful for a task, he jumped into action, keeping the doors from closing while I grabbed Wendi's wig and loose-fitting shirt from the floor. I hoisted her into my arms and moved toward the exit. He followed, still processing but now committed.

Two more doors. Keys in hand. I eventually got her to the car, and before opening the door and lowering her into the seat, I handed the keys off to him. "Passenger door," I instructed, calling out in a calm but direct manner.

He opened it. Held it. Hesitated. One more ask remained.

"Mind holding her up for a sec?"

And so, in a moment he surely hadn't anticipated when he started his day, this man found himself bracing a semiconscious, bald, topless woman, while I ran to the driver's side. As soon as I was in position, he let go. "Appreciate you," I called out, already shifting into gear.

He shut the door behind us. The last glimpse I had was him standing there, hands on his hips, staring after us, adjusting to the fact that our normal had just collided with his. And then we were gone, racing toward yet another ER visit, another bag of saline, another night in the fight.

Every descent starts somewhere. Ours began long before that door closed, back when normal still felt like something you could count on.

THE ALWAYS SLIDING DOOR OF NORMAL

By our mid-fifties, life felt like smooth sailing. I'd met my beautiful wife in college, and her boundless energy had carried us through every twist life tossed our way. A petite cheerleader at Washington State University, she had a way of looking at the world as if every moment offered something new, something worth diving into.

Not long after our wedding, she became the breadwinner—working two jobs while I clawed my way through law school. She poured her energy into work, remodeling our first home, and showing up consistently as a willing, tireless study partner during countless late-night cram sessions. Those sleep-deprived years forged a partnership that would quietly prepare us for much harder days to come. Whether we knew they were coming or not.

And Two Makes Three . . . Leading to Six

I didn't realize it at first, but with the birth of our first child, Wendi stepped so naturally into the role of CEO when it came to parenting—and I was more than fine being middle management. The "how-to" questions—how to warm a bottle, how to store breast milk, how to swaddle a newborn—landed squarely in her lap. Even the monumental shift from the freedom of young adulthood into the chaos of parenthood somehow became hers to carry, which she did without complaint.

As our family grew, so did our rhythm. Wendi led the way in raising each of our four children. She also built a remarkable network of friends—people who would raise kids alongside us, sharing middle age with us, and (spoiler alert) stand shoulder to shoulder when illness came for some of us. Her boundless energy never faded. She kept renovating homes with the same enthusiasm she brought to parenting. Her unwavering support of my career gave me the confidence to take risks, and her ability to greet every new chapter with childlike joy instilled in me a deep desire to honor and protect her—something I would later cling to with everything I had.

Early Stress (A.K.A. Child's Play)

Stress—real or imagined—never really takes a day off. Looking back, it's surprising how many "crisis" moments now seem trivial in hindsight. Yet, at the time we experienced them, they felt anything but. Closets rarely come without monsters lurking inside, and we're often the ones inadvertently feeding them. We imagine the worst, and in doing so, we give these monsters form, breath, and power. Even as we move through life and slay a few of these damn monsters, new ones take their place.

In calm moments, it's easy to recognize that the past wasn't as devastating as it once seemed, the present isn't as bleak as it feels, and the future isn't as uncertain as we fear. Easy to see—when you're not staring into the eyes of a freshly created monster.

The mind is a master storyteller. Left unchecked, it can build stress from thin air, like a snowball gathering speed down a hill. Don't believe it? Just think back.

When we were newly married, with fledgling careers and growing families, how did balancing a checkbook feel? Daunting? Hopeless? Somehow, we got through it, if only by a nickel or a dime.

And how did we cope with that self-inflicted stress? Lavish getaways? Vacation homes in Cabo? Not exactly. Our escape came through friendships—fellow monster-slayers living parallel lives. Most of the time, our "vacations" happened in cramped apartments, around a folding table, with a deck of cards. Those weekend afternoons and evenings were our defense. Our shield. And in many ways, our joy.

Evolution of Perspectives

Looking back on those early, formidable, and oh-so-stressful early years, it's amazing how many of them now feel . . . cherished. Everything was new. Expectations were modest. Apartments were smaller; so were bills—and paychecks. Life revolved around launching careers, raising babies, and learning how to be married. No one was terribly concerned with keeping up with the Joneses, as the Joneses were just starting out themselves. What once felt like overwhelming stress now looks a lot more like growth, even joy, in disguise.

Remember the game *Who Moves First*? If you're a parent and you claim you never played it, go see a priest and confess. You are full of shit.

This wasn't a game so much as a battle. It usually began with a faint cry in the middle of the night—just a slight whisper over the baby monitor on the nightstand. Ask either parent under oath, and they may both swear they didn't hear it. Let's chalk that up to innocent perjury. And as that cry grew louder and longer, both contestants in the game lay motionless, each silently praying the other would move first.

Once the cry gained energy—audible both from the monitor and down the hall—the game clock was officially ticking. Action needed to be taken. You could feel the tension rise with each wail. It was go time, but both contestants continued to remain motionless.

Now, for those blessed with multiple kids, the game came with advanced levels. Sometimes a contestant would emit a passive-aggressive sigh. Other times, more physical tactics may be used. By the time our fourth child arrived, Wendi's strategy evolved to utilizing a not-so-loving foot shoved into my back, which she deployed with increasing accuracy, helping to encourage my movement.

As the loser stumbled down the dark hallway to comfort a child, the victor rolled over to jump back into slumber, likely wearing a silent, satisfied grin. Of course, no one stayed undefeated for long. The game always reset, sometimes within the same night. But each blurry-eyed walk of shame to the crib offered the loser one undeniable consolation prize: guilt that could be leveraged in the next round.

And this—this silly, maddening ritual—shines a light on how perspective shifts and evolves so dramatically over time. Back then, it felt stressful. Exhausting. Now? I look back on those middle-of-the-night battles with a smile. With joy. Of course, that's easy for me to say. I remember having more wins than losses.

Life In the Now

Like many of our peers, we've been blessed with grandchildren—three so far, with more on the way. Though these babies currently live in Europe, we cross the pond whenever we can, cramming into a small apartment to soak up every moment. Clearly, technology has evolved. Today, baby monitors come with cameras and night vision. I noticed that when visiting my grandkids in Europe. What I also noticed is that the rules of *Who Moves First?* have not changed. At least for my daughter and son-in-law.

On the other hand, the game has shifted in meaningful ways for Wendi and me. The monitor now lives on the nightstand in our daughter's bedroom. While they certainly engage in the age-old standoff of parental endurance during those late-night battles, Wendi and I, tucked away in a quieter room, are playing an entirely new version.

When the first cry echoes through the apartment, we don't freeze. We race. Now it's not about who can stay motionless the longest; it has shifted to who can get to the grandbaby *first*. The same sound that once meant stress and sleeplessness now pulls us from bed with a kind of joy we never saw coming, at least for the first few nights of the visit.

By the end of the trip, when sleep deprivation begins to catch up, we quietly shift our strategy. As the cry builds steam, we both lie still, smiling, giggling, and silently cheering on our daughter as she enters a round of *Who Moves First?* with her husband.

Grandparent ears must be wired differently. The same cries, the same blurry nights. Only now, these cries land sweetly on the heart instead of pounding directly against the nerves.

The Future, Anyone?

Will there be monsters in the future? A resounding yes, as I can attest.

Big, hairy, raging ones. The closets may change, but the things that lurk inside? Still monsters. But just like grandparent ears hear a child's cry differently, our perspectives will continue to evolve.

Let's stay with the theme of *Who Moves First?*

We currently share our home with a little lap dog that our grown kids insist we cannot live without. Like most pampered poochers, she's earned full family status—and a permanent hall pass to sleep on our bed. That is, unless one of our kids is visiting. In that case, we're suddenly discarded like chopped liver while she curls up with them instead. Our poocher has made it clear she wouldn't have it any other way.

In our current home, there's a sliding glass door precisely fifty-three inches from Wendi's side of the bed. How can I be that precise? I have personally measured it. Often. Why? Strategy. After years in the trenches of *Who Moves First?*, I've learned that every inch counts.

Some nights, our spoiled little poocher hops off the bed, ready for a late-night visit to the backyard. The instant her paws hit the floor, the game is back on. As she trots toward the door and begins her ritual scratch on the glass, both contestants freeze, remaining motionless—seasoned veterans—each waiting for the other to flinch first.

No words are exchanged. None needed. The rules have not changed. The setting has. The players have. The time in our lives has. But the spirit of the game? Alive and well.

Besides visualizing the distance between Wendi and the sliding glass door, as a seasoned veteran in *Who Moves First?*, I've added a few signature moves for whenever I rise for the revised walk of shame. Maybe the door isn't closed as gently as it could be. Maybe a highly unnecessary light gets flipped on. Perhaps even left on. On these occasions when I make the walk of shame, the winning contestant—still motionless—wears a knowing smile, deeply enjoying her victory and my tactics. And her smile is stretching across those infuriating fifty-three inches.

It is amazing how "in the moment" evolves over time—how distance lets me look back and wonder why stress was ever allowed a front-row seat in our lives. Our game of "Who Moves First" captured that perfectly, a snapshot of the ever-changing moments of normalcy. In our younger years, the cries of a child pierced the night and soaked the mind in sleep-deprived self-pity. *Poor me* was the prevailing thought, as the loser shuffled toward a crib in the dark. As wins and losses are counted in the mind, a bit of anger is inevitable, normally carrying over to be used the next morning. It is almost pathetic how many needless arguments were born from those evenings, arguments playing out over the course of four children, night after night. Fast-forward to the same cries, now coming from a grandchild. And yet—an entirely different response from these same cries. A joyful sprint to be the first one to the crib. Same cries, now just received differently.

And when it is just the two of us, alone in the house, is normalcy now placing us in a quiet role of empty nesters? Nope. Game on. We're back to the battle, this time over a spoiled lap dog needing a midnight potty break. The game remains. But the tone has softened. In the morning, instead of grumbles or scorekeeping, the conversation turns playful. Teasing. Maybe even a tape measure comes out again, confirming—without leaving any doubt—that she's still fifty-three inches from the damn door.

That's the thing about perspective. It evolves. What once felt stressful now makes us laugh. What seemed urgent becomes endearing. Seemingly stressful events can appear so different when viewed in a rearview mirror. That is, until you are playing for keeps.

Whatever Normal Was, It Was No Longer

For most, the early spring of 2021 marked the first signs of a slow return toward normalcy, a normalcy that was shattered so abruptly for all. The previous March, in 2020, the US—along with much of the world—had shut down in response to the unknowns brought on by COVID. "Shelter at home" became more than a policy; it became a way of life. While these measures were an effort to reduce the spread of the virus, they also triggered something else: a pandemic-level surge in anxiety, depression, and mental fatigue. Social isolation crept in and settled deep. Mental health professionals scrambled as communities tried to dig out from a year unlike any other.

The lingering fog of that isolation stretched through the winter of 2020 and into early 2021. Then spring arrived. Which comes a bit earlier in Scottsdale, Arizona.

Blue skies, blooming trees, and bursts of color seemed to shout something the world desperately needed to hear: *Begin again.*

Spring always nudges us toward renewal, but this one felt particularly urgent. After more than a year of collective weariness and uncertainty, it finally felt like we were being given permission to breathe again. Live again.

For us, one date was circled on the calendar and stood out—a weekend that felt like it could mark the beginning of something better. Some of our closest friends and loved ones were coming down to Scottsdale for a visit. A *real visit.* The first real visit (not a Zoom call) in what felt like forever. We highlighted that date on the calendar with hope and excitement. The weather delivered, the company was perfect, and what unfolded wasn't just a visit. It was a celebration.

We golfed. We laughed. We retold pandemic bunker stories and toasted the simple fact that we were together again. Okay. Maybe too many glasses were lifted, but even that somehow made it all more perfect.

None of us believed, coming out of that weekend, that normal was fully restored. But that weekend? That first weekend together? It was a massive step in the right direction.

When they returned to Boise, we felt blessed—and eager. Eager to build on the momentum toward a new normalcy. Eager to keep reaching toward the version of life we all missed so much.

We had no idea that while we were still basking in the glow of that visit, the ground beneath us was already beginning to shift. And not in the way we hoped or could have imagined.

For us, what came next wasn't a step forward. It also wasn't just a step backward. It was a total collapse.

What an Unexpected Gut Punch Feels Like

Just as winter was loosening its grip and we were easing into that early, hopeful stretch of spring, Wendi found a lump on her left breast. It was late January 2021. I remember how calmly she picked up the phone, how matter-of-factly she described it to her healthcare provider in Boise. Because of the post-COVID backlog still clogging the system, they told her to simply mention this during her mammogram the following month.

February arrived, and with it a routine appointment that became anything but. The mammogram led to more questions, then more images, and before we fully understood what was happening, an ultrasound was scheduled for early March. The pace wasn't frantic, but it was steady, like a current pulling us somewhere neither of us wanted to go.

The timing of the visit from our Boise friends was ideal, as it allowed us to stay grounded in the ordinary. I remember a few of the women gently asking Wendi if she'd heard anything back from the tests. Wendi would just shrug, offer a quick smile, and pull herself back into the moment, doing everything she could to keep the weight of the unknown from landing too soon.

March 5, 2021

What we didn't know was that when the gut punch came, it wouldn't be one clean blow. Rather, it would come in parts. Part one landed in the most familiar, safe space in our home: the kitchen counter. On an otherwise normal Friday afternoon, Wendi's phone rang. I happened to be sitting next to her when she picked up the call. I couldn't hear the voice on the other end, but I didn't need to. Her face said it all. Something was terribly wrong.

My instinct on reading her face was spot-on. The call was short, but its impact was massive. The test results showed that she had breast cancer. Gut punch, part one. Delivered and felt, right there, at our kitchen counter.

There wasn't much information provided, just the call with the words that everyone fears. The call that no one is ever truly prepared to receive. But in that single moment, three things happened that would change our lives forever.

First, the nurse's voice gave us an abrupt introduction to a world we didn't know we were about to enter—a world of scan results, oncology consults, new terminology, and learning on the fly.

Second, Wendi had just joined a sorority no one ever asks to join, but it's one filled with extraordinary, compassionate souls: women who had faced the demon known as breast cancer and who wear the pink ribbon not as decoration but as a badge of both survival and strength. Having faced this common enemy, these women are bound together and, on demand, eager to lift each other up in so many ways. I've come to admire that pink ribbon deeply. I often refer to this incredible sisterhood as the Pink Ribbon Brigade. Following that gut punch of a phone call, Wendi became a ribbon-carrying member, ready or not.

And third, I was suddenly—instantly—cast into a role I had never trained for: caregiver. Much like becoming a father for the first time or entering a marriage following a honeymoon, it is a baton you pick up and run with, experience be damned. At that moment, I didn't yet understand just how completely that role would change me. Forever.

No Good Way to Deliver Bad News

I can only imagine how difficult it must be for healthcare providers to find the right words when they are forced to deliver a gut punch to an unsuspecting patient. In our case, gut punch number one came fast—and with very little context. After dropping the "C" word into our lives, the nurse scheduled a follow-up call with Wendi's doctor for the following Monday.

That left us with a long weekend filled with shock, fear, and uncertainty.

I'm not sure if this is standard protocol—this was, after all, experience number one of one—but on the surface, it made some sense. We received the immediate, disorienting blow, and then we were given a pause. A chance to absorb, to brace, to begin processing this new reality before stepping into the details of diagnosis and treatment.

That weekend was a blur of quiet moments—long stares, a few tears, and an overwhelming amount of silence. Neither of us knew what to say. And so, we said very little.

There's no instruction manual for this kind of thing, but I did manage to land on one early decision. I gently urged Wendi not to tell anyone. Not yet. Not until we knew more. We're fortunate to have an incredible circle of friends and loved ones, people who have celebrated milestones with us and raised kids alongside us, lovely souls who would surely drop everything to rally around Wendi. They would absolutely want to know. They would absolutely want to help. But I felt strongly that we should wait. That we only share once we had something real to say, more than just pushing fear and uncertainty along. We needed a diagnosis. A plan. A way forward. And until then, we would hold this quietly, just the two of us.

And most certainly, we would share with loved ones *only* after our adult children knew.

Having made the decision to stay quiet, we found ourselves with just one thing on our minds that weekend: the scheduled call on Monday. Tick. Tick. Tick.

My pacing habit—perfected during COVID—picked up steam that weekend. As I wandered through the house and our neighborhood, eager to burn off nervous energy, I noticed something else: our loyal little poocher, Winter, a King Charles cavalier, absolutely refused to leave Wendi's side. Not for a second. She knew something was off. She always did.

While the nurse gave us almost no details during that brief call, she did offer one piece of advice that turned out to be invaluable. She gently urged us not to dive into the internet. And while everything in us wanted immediacy in answers, that advice stuck. Looking back, I'm so grateful we listened.

We knew so little. And the internet, with its infinite rabbit holes and worst-case scenarios, would have only amplified our fears. That weekend was already saturated with anxiety and uncertainty—why throw gasoline on the fire? As tempting as it was to start searching, we resisted. We stayed in the not-knowing, hard as it was.

There would be time for googling and planning. But not yet. Not before we had something more tangible to work with. No need to start the "what-if" game before the game had even begun.

TNBC

Even the really shitty forms of cancer come with acronyms.

As we counted down toward the Monday call, TVs ran unwatched, and silent stares filled the passing minutes. But pass they did, and eventually, we arrived at the first of many breath-hold moments ahead.

When the call with the doctor came, Wendi put on her brave face, instinctively grabbed a pen and notebook, and sat at the counter (yes, that same kitchen counter) as I watched—stoic, silent, helpless—as a conversation unfolded that no one is truly prepared for.

One thing became clear during that call: The simple act of holding a pen made a difference. Writing things down calmed her nerves. More importantly, it helped capture details that stress might have otherwise erased. That notebook became more than a tool—it became a shield, a place to store facts too heavy to carry in the moment, and a way to manage the sadness, anger, and fear that would undoubtedly surface. There would be time for the emotions to spill out later. During that call, we had to listen. And absorb.

Looking back at those notes, we were told Wendi had multiple tumors in her left breast. One of them was large enough to place her at Stage 2. We also heard, for the first time, the name of a rare form of breast cancer: triple-negative breast cancer. Yup. You guessed it. TNBC. At that point, TNBC meant very little—other than the word "rare," which landed hard.

Triple-negative breast cancer is diagnosed through a tissue analyzed in a pathology lab, where they look at three receptors: estrogen, progesterone, and HER2. By that Monday, Wendi had tested negative for two of these receptors. We were still waiting for results on the third. And apparently, this is one of those times in medicine when a "negative" result is not what you're hoping for.

The doctor didn't spend much time on the nuances of TNBC, but his tone said enough. We were cheering against receiving a third negative result.

He then encouraged us to reach out to an oncologist and start booking consultations. Once the word "oncologist" entered the conversation, it was clear that no matter how the third test turned out, our lives had already changed. Breast cancer had taken its place at the center of our story. Normal was about to shift yet again.

And just like that, the second gut punch landed—deep, hard, and impossible to ignore.

The Hardest Phone Call Ever Placed

After we hung up, the certainty absorbed, it was time for real tears to flow. And while I held her, telling her everything would be all right, my mind was racing as I knew those were merely words. We sat in the kitchen for a while, staring at one another, both with absolutely zero experience as to what comes next. As the tears slowed, an innate instinct kicked in, knowing she needed strength and leadership. She had taken a few gut punches as of late. Time to step up and act.

As brutally painful as it was going to be, step one was to bring our four adult children in on the news. They needed to hear this first and certainly directly from us. I did not recognize it at the time, but with this first decision, my former normal was being abruptly left behind and an eighteen-month journey as primary caregiver had just quietly commenced.

While my wife summoned some strength, I grabbed my phone and texted our four kids, whereabouts unknown, letting them know we needed a group FaceTime. ASAP. Having never sent a text like that previously, I am sure each of my kids' minds raced toward all different kinds of rabbit holes.

At the time, one kid was still in college in Oregon, one kid lived in Northern California, one was living in Boise, and our fourth and oldest was living overseas. Spread out as they were, it took some time to group together, even with the ASAP text. The texts were flying, our more communicative kids wanting immediate answers. I held off, believing they deserved to hear this news together. Strength in numbers.

Once my son's basketball practice ended, it was go time. I saw the panic across my children's faces, and it was absolutely killing me to deliver this news. No reason to delay or make small talk. They knew something bad was coming. They could see it as clear as day. "Guys, your mom and I love you very much, and as a family, we need to rally together," I started. Pause. Breathe. And then I said it. "Your Mom has breast cancer." Shock. Disbelief. Fear. All the emotions you do not want to see on the faces of your kids.

Saying it out loud for the first time made it real, and in no time, the tears were flowing. For all of us. Once the tears began to subside, the questions came from all of them. Looking back, it is amazing how very little we knew at the time of the hardest call ever made. The questions lost steam as the kids realized answers were not coming. At first, they may have thought we were holding back. Eventually, they gave up and, I am sure, started turning to google for the answers. What I desperately wanted to convey to the kids was that Mom had been so damn strong over the years, holding this family up and together. Now it was our turn to be strong for her. And, yes, hold her up. As I repeated this plea, I realized my kids had witnessed something they had rarely seen over the years. Dad was crying. A lot.

This realization led me to make a decision: I would hold back on future tears until after her treatment was complete. Here I was, asking my kids to be strong for Mom. For me, it went deeper than that. I felt the need to exhibit strength for my wife, my kids, our friends, and our loved ones. I realized my reaction, from this point forward, would be closely read for clues. I suddenly felt that displaying strength would breed strength, and I inherently knew that strength would become such a critical element through this uncharted journey. While unanticipated individual challenges were indeed realized later, I stand by this decision and believe that displaying strength provided strength. Even at the risk of causing mental trauma after treatment is complete.

A Family Goes All In, Together

Once we hung up, I left Wendi for a minute and started individual dialogues with the kids. These were young adults, either starting careers or finishing college. One was a young mother herself. They were also coming off the mental challenges of the COVID lockdowns and were all desperately seeking a return to normalcy. In their case, the return to normalcy took an unexpected turn.

My goal with these individual calls was to assess their personal reaction and provide some strength to each. My son wanted to quit school and hoops and return home. Understandable, but nope. He easily and quickly understood that this is not what Mom would want. Other offers of support flowed in from the girls. When I hung up from these individual calls, I could not have been prouder as a parent. The speed and manner in which they absorbed this shocking news and began rallying to their mother's side was a thing of pure beauty. I am so happy that we started delivering the news of Wendi's diagnosis to our "inner" circle. Through us or through others, the news would surely widen soon enough. By starting small, a circle of strength was formed that was desperately needed. Love, strength, and support would come from expected and unexpected sources throughout the journey. But as the bumps and bruises along the way piled up, an inner circle of strength was so critical to rely upon, whether merely to vent or to use as a communication tool during a changing normalcy. Consistent reliance on an inner circle definitely helps to stay in the game, particularly when you are playing on fumes.

Here Comes the Pink Ribbon Brigade

While I was talking with the kids individually, Wendi and her loyal poocher retreated to our bedroom. From there, she started seeking out strength and support by informing her close friends and loved ones. These initial calls exposed her to the Pink Ribbon Brigade. This informal group is an extremely tight, protective, loving group of individuals that eagerly and unselfishly look to pay it forward. They compassionately talk about their experiences and offer resources for the uneducated just starting their journey.

As Wendi dialed her friends, many had a friend or someone they knew who had previously been placed on the breast cancer journey. These calls led to more calls, usually culminating in a conversation with a previous stranger, an individual within the Pink Ribbon Brigade, willing to share experiences, resources, and advice. In those early hours, days, and weeks, where every day felt new and our previous normalcy was quickly fading away, this support network of breast cancer survivors, most of whom she had never met, provided her with great comfort knowing she was not alone. Strength in numbers again. I will forever be grateful for these nurturing souls who so unselfishly offered their time and support. Particularly in those early moments, when up is down, left is right, and nothing feels normal, the Pink Ribbon Brigade enters your life and makes a massive impact. Kudos, ladies. Your staircase to heaven is being built.

Time to Fight-or-Flight

While Wendi spent the days ahead healing and gaining strength through numbers, diving deep into the Pink Ribbon Brigade, I never felt more alone. Friends, having no shared experiences, didn't know what to say, so they mostly stayed away. I felt myself quickly retreating into a fight-or-flight mindset. As fear or danger is perceived, the mind is trained to use its resources to keep us safe. The Cleveland Clinic identifies four main responses to stress or fear that can be triggered when entering fight-or-flight: 1) Duh. Fight; 2) Again, duh. Flight (thanks, Cleveland Clinic); 3) Freeze; and 4) Fawn. Nothing too earth-shattering here, as the first three are quite obvious in both their definition and approach. The fourth refers to a tactic where the individual attempts to appease or reconcile the threat in order to find protection. Without offering a specific plan, your mind assesses the danger and determines the options that best provide safety.

While I did not fully grasp this at the time, I fell deeply into fight-or-flight mode. Following the initial gut punch, this protective instinct took over for me and lasted eighteen months. Eighteen months . . .

The duration of this mentality, while beneficial within our evolving day-to-day normalcy, did not come without unintended side effects. One identified side effect, particularly when fight-or-flight becomes a prolonged behavioral tool, is (spoiler alert) that memories can be impacted. More on this later.

With Wendi graciously accepting the love and support of the Pink Ribbon Brigade, my mind, fully mired in fight-or-flight, instinctually selected the "fight" option as its chosen method to combat our danger. I suddenly felt an urge to assert some level of control over our new path. This started with taking control of a calendar. While my wife's physician said he would reach out to an oncologist to make a referral, no timetable was provided. I needed more. Working the phone, I began sourcing out resources within the medical community. This initial chain of calls, with so little information to offer at the time, did lead us to a list of oncologists in our former hometown of Boise. Step one. Having names in hand, my fight instinct took over. I began calling in favors, something I'd rarely done, and never for myself. Calendars were booked, but I kept dialing, likely wearing out patience and burning through goodwill I'd spent years building in Boise. Still, the calls mattered. Within days, we were heading north—appointments secured with an oncologist and an oncology surgeon in Boise, both coming highly recommended.

What we couldn't have known at the time was that every hour mattered. Moving fast felt like the right thing to do for emotional stability—finding a path to answers, to a plan. But it turned out to be much more than that.

We later learned that from the time Wendi first felt the lump in January to the start of chemo treatment in March, her cancer had already progressed from stage 1 to stage 2.

Turns out, hours counted. Every one of them.

Cutting the Line

Everything moved faster than I thought possible. Relationships tended and nurtured over the years now shifted calendars, opened doors, and turned waiting weeks into days. For the first time since her diagnosis, we weren't standing still. We were moving—driven, unrelenting, searching for a way forward. Neither of us had ever been the type to press this hard, but that shift in posture, that decision to lean forward instead of waiting, likely saved her life.

Before we could blink, we were landing in Boise. Upon hitting the tarmac, I'd already made a firm decision: I would be absolutely pinned to Wendi's side every step of the way, my fear of hospitals be damned. She would need support through this unfamiliar storm, and the best way I could offer this was to stand shoulder to shoulder with her—as the uneducated became educated.

Landing in Boise felt different this time. The comfort of what used to be home did not cushion the unease. It was as if an extremely familiar city had been draped in something new and foreign. We were about to meet people we'd never known, discuss things we barely understood, and visit places in Boise never previously seen. Boise, once our grounding point, was no longer a refuge. It quickly became the threshold of something unknown. And scary.

Without knowing what we were about to walk into, the first oncologist we met delivered yet another gut punch.

We'd heard of triple-negative breast cancer, and we knew there was still one test result pending—the third receptor. According to him, unfortunately, the wait for this test result was over.

Time to admit it: Before we left for Boise, I had finally ignored the nurse's advice and dipped a toe deep into the internet rabbit hole to perform some TNBC research. I didn't get far, but I did get far enough to realize we did not want the third test result to be negative.

After a brief exam, feeling her lumps, oncologist number one launched into a description of his preferred treatment path for TNBC. That was the moment it hit me like a runaway freight train. Gut punch number three landed: an unexpected but now confirmed diagnosis of TNBC.

He had no idea we hadn't yet been told. No idea that his calm, clinical delivery of TNBC treatment options was doubling as our introduction to a life-altering reality. Wendi had TNBC, a rare and aggressive form of invasive cancer, found in only about 15 percent of all cases. As he continued in his matter-of-fact tone, my head began to spin with terminology I'd never heard before.

It's strange how even when your world shifts violently, little things can still cut deep. Wendi didn't know it at the time, but I mentally scratched oncologist number one off our list before we even left the room. Not for what he said, nor for how he said it. We understood so little then; most of his words flew right over our heads.

No, it was the little things that did it. And they still mattered, even now.

As is probably standard protocol, our meeting began with a quick breast exam. But what followed surprised me. He went straight into his detailed explanation of treatment options—never pausing, never offering, never allowing Wendi a moment to cover back up. She heard the words "triple-negative breast cancer" and sat there, exposed and vulnerable, through the entire conversation.

He may not have noticed. But I sure did. And that was enough. Little things still matter, even as previous normalcy fades away.

Life So Rarely Slows

We spent that first evening in Boise trying to process what we'd just learned: Wendi had TNBC. She retreated to her room, immersing herself in conversations with members of her newly discovered sorority—women who had walked this road before her. Through that Pink Ribbon Brigade network, she eventually connected with others who had received this same rare diagnosis. There was a real comfort for Wendi in speaking directly to those within that 15 percent.

Meanwhile, I descended further into fight-or-flight mode, slamming my phone into action as I cast a wider net in search of oncologists and a treatment plan. I began looking everywhere—Houston, Southern California, Seattle. My focus was singular: the best possible care, delivered with absolute urgency.

In my shallow dive into the world of TNBC, two phrases had branded themselves into my mind. The first was the term "rare." And in my untrained thinking, "rare" meant we needed to look for care in places where cutting-edge research was being conducted. The second phrase? Fast-growing cells. That one dug even deeper. Given her cancer was already Stage 2 and her cells were being classified as fast-growing, my instincts screamed that immediacy mattered.

Oddly, I expected time to slow. That's what you'd assume when your world narrows and hyperfocus takes over. But instead, time just kept barreling forward. Even as our schedules were cleared, the days came at us faster. And in the blink of an eye, we were sitting in front of the first oncology surgeon we had ever met.

Within a few moments, we both felt more at ease. Some of the shock had worn off by then, but her approach helped too. Like the first appointment in Boise, she began with a brief breast exam—but then she paused, looked at Wendi, and asked her to get dressed before continuing the conversation. A small gesture, sure. But to us, it meant everything. Little things still mattered.

As she walked us through her recommended treatment plan, the differences were clear. Her words were calm, considered. This wasn't her first case of TNBC, but it was our first anything. She didn't rush. She gave us space to breathe, to catch up, to learn.

And we learned a lot in that meeting. We discovered the distinction between an oncologist (the one responsible for the treatment path) and an oncology surgeon (the surgeon who will remove the tumors and, potentially, some or all of the breast tissue). New terms were delivered. Neoadjuvant chemotherapy, meaning chemotherapy would be administered before surgery to shrink the tumors and improve surgical outcomes. This was the oncology surgeon's preferred approach to address TNBC. We also heard that surgery would include lymph node removal or harvesting, which would help assess potential cancer cell spread.

Her tone and approach were very different from the oncologist we had met with, but her recommended treatment plan was surprisingly similar. That gave us a quiet sense of reassurance. Maybe we were beginning to understand the road ahead.

We left this meeting feeling cautiously hopeful—except for one glaring exception. She wanted to begin treatment in sixty days.

Maybe it was a scheduling issue. Maybe it was typical protocol. But to someone running on pure adrenaline, deep in fight-or-flight mode, and haunted by the word "fast-growing," sixty days felt like an eternity. I was still a novice in all of this, but in my gut, I couldn't make that timeline make any sense.

Back to the Drawing Board

We left Boise with a clearer sense of direction regarding a path forward, but still with nothing concrete on the calendar. *Fast-growing cells* had been resonating in my head ever since we received informal confirmation of TNBC. I was desperately searching for a date I could place on the calendar, getting this treatment path started. And so I continued to work the phones, continued to look for care facilities that also conducted research.

Now that we were living in the Scottsdale area for part of the year, the Mayo Clinic certainly came to mind. That being said, I naively viewed the Mayo Clinic as a mysterious place, a type of castle on the hill that required some form of a Willy Wonka Golden Ticket to gain admission. Golden Ticket be damned, the Mayo Clinic was twenty minutes from my house, and I was in full fight mode. Not knowing the rules of engagement, I set my sights solely on gaining admission into this castle on the hill.

Lots of phone time and pleading taught me that Mayo was insurance-friendly, affiliated with our main hospital back in Boise, and potentially accessible. In my current state of mind, however, being *potentially* accessible was not good enough. I desperately needed it to be *immediately* accessible. More phone time. More leads. Some dead ends. Eventually, the hours spent on the phone did pay off, and I was able to find the golden ticket for which I had been desperately searching. Through relatives and friends, we eventually found an individual outside of Mayo who had a contact inside of Mayo, and hearing of Wendi's diagnosis, Mayo Oncology scheduled an appointment. Within days of arriving back from Boise, we were walking into the mysterious castle on the hill with the words *Mayo Clinic* on top.

The Castle on the Hill

We didn't know it until after we checked in, but Mayo did not schedule *an* appointment with us. Rather, Mayo scheduled a series of back-to-back appointments for us. After our mandatory COVID tests were complete and negative, we checked in and realized we would be at Mayo for a while. We would start with an oncologist, followed by an oncology surgeon, and then finish our day with a reconstructive surgeon. While not knowing what to expect, we gained comfort in being able to talk with a healthcare team to help us catch up to our new normal.

Some initial impressions with the previously mysterious Mayo Clinic are as follows: First, they are much more community-oriented than I had previously believed. Second, they happily accepted insurance and, more importantly, my form of insurance. Finally, the professionalism we experienced from the first moment we entered those mysterious halls was off the charts. While the quality of care our family had enjoyed during our thirty years in the Boise community was fantastic, the professionalism and approach of the Mayo Clinic was nothing like I had ever experienced before.

From the moment we walked in, we were never alone. Upon completing check-in, we were led to meet our oncology PA, who would also serve as our personal concierge throughout our appointments scheduled for that day. She dutifully stayed by our side for all of our appointments and for the moments in between, willingly prepared to answer any questions that we generated during our whirlwind of a day.

Oncologist, Mayo Style

One more element that differentiated Mayo from prior experience. Appointments started on time. Again, even in our new normal, little things matter. Our meeting with the oncologist at Mayo started punctually and, once again, began with a brief breast examination. Upon completion of this examination, the oncologist left the room while Wendi got redressed.

Upon his return, we realized that Mayo had received all imaging records from Boise. Even better, all the caregivers we met with that day had taken the time to study her charts and imaging results before our meetings. Our Mayo oncologist handed us a treatment notebook and paperwork describing his recommended treatment path and steps forward, in depth. As he walked us through each step, he encouraged us to take notes and patiently paused for our questions. Here are the notes we were able to take during that initial discussion:

- Two types of chemotherapy would be administered every week for twelve weeks.
- Two different types of chemotherapy would be administered following these initial twelve weeks. These different types would be administered a total of four times, every other week.

- After a period to allow the body an appropriate time for recovery, surgery would occur to remove any remaining tumors, including breast tissue around the margins of the tumors. Some lymph nodes would be harvested to test for any potential spread.
- In the event Wendi elects to proceed with a single or double mastectomy, this would be performed at the time of surgery.
- *Finally* (breathe), depending on Wendi's decision regarding mastectomy or how much tissue would need to be removed around margins, breast reconstruction of some form would be scheduled and performed on the same day following the work completed by the oncology surgeon.

The information did not stop there. We not only received a specific treatment path that day, but we also began hearing chemo terms for the very first time. Again, referring to our notes from that first meeting, the types of chemo that would be administered were detailed as follows:

- For the initial twelve weeks of weekly chemo treatments, Wendi would be receiving paclitaxel, a.k.a. Taxol, and carboplatin, a.k.a. Paraplatin.
- For the biweekly treatments (weeks twelve to twenty), Wendi would be receiving cyclophosphamide, a.k.a. Cytoxan, and, finally, doxorubicin, a.k.a. Rubex, or the Red Devil.
- Per my hope to find a treatment center that engages heavily in research, the doctor also mentioned that, if Wendi were to qualify and had an interest, near the end of her chemo treatments, she could be eligible for a study they were conducting. In this case, she would receive pembrolizumab, a.k.a. Keytruda, which is used in cancer immunotherapy.

Wow. Typing this out from our notes, that was certainly a lot to digest. With all the timelines and new terms, our minds were racing and swimming in new data points. Crazy as it sounds, these were notes taken from our first of three meetings that day, with different care providers. While I recall the feeling of being overwhelmed with data, I also recall feeling somewhat calm, knowing we were hearing a very specific path forward.

Although we were indeed hearing a path, we were still lacking a schedule. After exhausting our questions, the calendar came next. No notes necessary. After reiterating that her cancer cells were fast-growing, which is part of TNBC, the doctor launched into a description of Wendi's specific tumors. He explained that her diagnosis of Stage 2 was a result of the largest of these tumors. Because of this and her TNBC diagnosis, he wanted to start treatments next week. On Monday. As in five days away.

We would both later describe how calming that was. The wait would be over. Action would happen, and the action would be near immediate.

We then heard about a chemo port for the first time. While optional, the oncologist was strongly encouraging this. Wendi, obviously hearing some input and suggestions from her newfound community of knowledgeable souls, seemed to understand what he was talking about. I had absolutely no clue. The port was a way to simplify the blood draws and chemo infusion by accessing a port as opposed to battling veins. Given Wendi's aggressive treatment schedule, he felt this would definitely increase her comfort. Wendi, having done pre-research on the topic, agreed. Unfortunately, because he wanted to begin treatments in five days, the minor surgery necessary to install the port could not be accomplished for seven to ten days. She would have to move forward with treatment without the aid of the port.

Oncology Surgeon

With all this information to absorb, the oncologist left us to our thoughts. While our heads were clearly spinning with these data points, a calmness was seeping into the room. Like clockwork, another oncology surgeon entered our lives. Shortly after she walked in, we both knew we would like her and would want to lean in with her. After sitting down near us, she turned her computer screen toward us, and, for the first time, we were staring at Wendi's tumors. One was larger than the other. She had circled these nasty bastards on the screen, describing them in both medical terms and layman's terms. Her description provided some clarity as to why we were about to embark upon the chemotherapy journey.

Because of Wendi's TNBC diagnosis, traditional hormone therapies and HER2-targeted drugs were off the table, as these would be ineffective. This narrowed treatment options considerably. She reiterated that the cells were fast-growing, which is why she agreed with starting treatment as fast as possible. She then walked us through the plan in its entirety, explaining it in very simple terms. Hearing it again, from a different source, certainly helped to allow it to truly sink in.

Beginning Monday, we were going to dive straight into the world of chemotherapy. These drugs and this treatment are intended to cease growth and, hopefully, shrink tumors, making the surgeon's job easier. While the imaging did not show any signs of spread beyond the left breast, she would harvest some lymph nodes during surgery and use them to help ensure there had been no further spread. Once the tumors are removed during surgery, the goal is to have clear, negative margins around the area formerly occupied by the tumors.

While still playing catch-up, the game plan was making a hell of a lot more sense: chemo to stop the growth and shrink tumors, surgery to remove tumors and the tissue around where the tumors grew, and lymph node harvesting to assess whether spread has occurred. Okay. Hands in the middle. Ready. Set. Go.

The severity of what lay ahead was explained to us in the clearest, bluntest terms our oncology surgeon could offer. On St. Patty's Day, mind you, by an oncology surgeon who was Irish.

TNBC didn't leave much room for nuance, she said. Options were limited, and the viable path forward was to hit it with everything modern medicine had. In her words, the treatment path was the equivalent of throwing the kitchen sink at it.

For us, that translated into an aggressive, unrelenting chemotherapy schedule, followed by surgery—a full-force approach meant to overwhelm the tumors before they overwhelmed her.

But wait. We had more to discuss. This discussion had a lean toward life after treatment, something we had not thought much about after the initial gut punch. Wendi had some choices to make. I insert Wendi here as the sole decision maker for good reason. While I have long admired her body since initially meeting her in college, it was nonetheless *her* body. Her body, her choice.

Our oncology surgeon began the discussion by laying out her options. Given the location of the tumors and because the tumors were only located in one breast, numerous options were available. Door number one was breast-conserving surgery, referred to as a lumpectomy. While not the preferred path for TNBC patients, it was nonetheless an option discussed. How much tissue the surgeon would have to take around the tumors would ultimately decide what kind of breast reconstruction, if any, could be done. Because tissue was being removed from only one breast, the surgeon's post-treatment goal was for the breasts to appear symmetrical. I saw relief in the oncology surgeon's face when Wendi quickly dismissed this option. Wendi had clearly done her homework and discussed this with her newfound support network within the Pink Ribbon Brigade. Wendi decisively ruled out door number one.

The discussion next moved toward a mastectomy, a term I knew very little about other than the implications. This meant the removal of all the breast tissue. While clearly Wendi had internally and previously made this decision, I was happy a discussion ensued so I could better understand what this all meant.

Because the cancerous cells existed in just one of her breasts,

Wendi had to decide whether to have a single or double mastectomy. After hearing her options, Wendi did not hesitate. Double. Remove all breast tissue. While she had clearly been given advice from her newfound support network, the promptness of this decision led me to believe that her conviction on this came from research and prayer. Her body. Her call. Done.

The surgeon felt obligated, I assume, to describe the slow and painful recovery associated with this major surgery, but upon hearing this, Wendi did not blink. I kept my eyes on the oncology surgeon throughout this discussion regarding surgical options. Much like a passenger on a plane during heavy turbulence, watching the flight attendant's reaction for reassurance, I was closely monitoring the surgeon's reactions to Wendi's decisions. Whether I was reading it correctly or not, I certainly felt reassured that the surgeon quietly agreed with Wendi's strong convictions.

There was still more to discuss, giving me little time to adjust to our ever-changing normal and the fact that my wife had just decided on a double mastectomy. I was now a party to a discussion regarding nipple-sparing surgery. How our normal had changed. Again, because of the size and location of the tumors, our surgeon could apparently remove all the breast tissue while preserving the skin, nipple, and areola. Damn. If my head was not spinning before, it sure was during that discussion.

I thought of a John Travolta and Nicholas Cage movie, where each of their faces was surgically removed and swapped to the other person. It was definitely a surreal feeling, listening to a discussion of nipple-sparing surgery, involving my wife, who seemed so damn healthy just weeks ago. I found myself thinking, for the first time since the initial gut punch, about life after treatment. Over time, I realized how important it was to picture a future beyond the fight—particularly in those moments when hope felt like a rare visitor.

Once Wendi opted for nipple-sparing surgery, the surgeon's discussion points were exhausted. But she could sense that we were still playing catch-up, and she gave no impression that we were on the clock. Rather, she sat patiently and compassionately, answering our many questions. Mostly coming from me. I asked about the chemo port, frankly, because I could not understand what the hell it was. She was an extremely visual person, so she drew a picture for me. It is a small reservoir inserted just below the skin in the chest area. A catheter tube coming from the port is then attached to a large vein, normally near the heart. This small device provides healthcare providers easy and quick access for blood draws, chemotherapy and IV-administered medication. It also reduces the discomfort for Wendi by reducing the need for multiple needle insertions over time. The surgeon went on to describe the cons: potential for clotting, infection, and the physical discomfort of living with a port inserted in your chest. I describe this only to emphasize how compassionate this individual was. This was certainly not her first rodeo, but it was definitely ours.

As she completed her port discussion, she pulled up her computer and gave us the date the port would be inserted. It was happening like clockwork. After leaving us earlier, the oncologist had already begun scheduling things for Wendi. What we could not have known at the time was that the chemo port, over the course of her treatment, would be used more than a television remote. Having to use needles and forcing medical providers to locate willing veins would certainly add stress to an already stressful situation. The port would prove to be a Godsend.

Blueprints for Tomorrow

Our questions exhausted, our oncology surgeon left the room. Although we didn't know it at the time, we would not see her or speak to her again for thirty weeks. We stayed behind in the room, feeling much more educated in our path. Before long, the door opened for a third time, and in walked a breast reconstruction surgeon. For the first time since the initial gut punch, someone was entering our lives to talk about something other than cancer. After weeks of hearing what needed to be taken, we were finally talking about what might be restored. It wasn't about vanity; it was about recovery, about imagining a body and a life that could somehow feel whole again.

Many moons prior, while living in our previous normal, my wife had considered cosmetic surgery for breast implants. I remember those conversations in our mid-thirties, mentally picturing my beautiful, petite wife stretching out the fabric in a nightgown or bikini just a bit further. Whatever my opinions were at that time (and I will forever take the fifth on that), my wife ultimately elected not to have the surgery. Her body. Her choice.

Some twenty years later, we were back again, discussing breast reconstruction, obviously under much different circumstances. While he obviously knew the circumstances, he talked in a way that made us feel thirty again. And without cancer in our lives. While our normal had changed, during these discussions, he was doing his part in shifting us to a time where the cancerous cells had been removed, where we would be shifting, once again, to a different normal. A cancer-free normal. This was a discussion I didn't want to end.

While I was still bracing for a double mastectomy in our future, Wendi and the surgeon were already talking about what could be rebuilt. I couldn't yet see that far ahead, but their words sketched the faint outline of a finish line. That is powerful imagery during such uncertain and confusing times. Looking back, I cannot accurately count how many times I reflected on this conversation and relied upon this imagery to help provide both strength and hope while we were in the middle of the grind.

My involvement in those reconstruction discussions was minimal, partly because I struggled to think that distantly. As a result, my notes from that meeting were thin at best. I understood that the reconstruction surgeon would step in as the oncology surgeon was finishing up, making for one long day in the OR. Then, assuming margins and lymph nodes cooperated, he would begin the delicate work of putting her back together again.

Because of the location of her tumors and her decision for a double mastectomy, she was a good candidate for implants, should she select that route. If she were to elect a larger size of saline or silicone implant, tissue expanders would need to be placed under the skin to help expand the area. This may also require multiple surgeries. Given that she had elected not to move forward with breast augmentation while in her mid-thirties, it did not surprise me when she quickly moved the conversation toward the fastest, most simplistic path. She had no interest in multiple surgeries and wanted to minimize post-surgery recovery time. He offered an option that would include the insertion of an implant in both breasts, similar in size to her existing breasts. This would eliminate the need for expanders. She latched on to that quickly.

She was pleased to hear that this could happen in one surgery. While there were many unknowns that he could not predict, he showed confidence that this would be the quickest path, and if she wanted additional changes down the road, she could opt for adjustments or cosmetic changes later. She continued to show conviction that she would be one and done and would opt to live with the cosmetic results. The way she had made such quick decisions that day, I believed her.

During this entire process, medical advancements would never cease to amaze me. Cold caps, which are exactly as the name describes, are placed on the head during chemo treatments to help reduce hair loss. Mayo offered this. Wendi declined. Along these lines, the reconstruction surgeon offered Wendi an alternative to implants. Called flap surgery, tissue is harvested from other parts of the body (normally the stomach, back, or lower buttocks), and this is used to rebuild the breast in lieu of an implant. Given what Wendi was going through, she was intrigued; foreign objects being inserted into her posttreatment did not sound *bueno* at the time. But when she next heard that flap surgery would require longer surgical time and, likely, longer recovery time, her interest began to fade quickly. She also did not like the sound of additional scarring in the areas from where the tissue was harvested. Let's be clear. This is a deeply personal decision with no right answer. And the decision is being made after a traumatic gut punch, as normalcy is changing rapidly. Wendi's focus was clearly on simplicity and a faster recovery time. She made the decision, on the spot, to have reconstruction using implants, sized in a manner that would not require expanders. Check the box.

One note here. While I did not record it in my notes, they did discuss not taking any action and opting instead for a flat closure. That option would come with even faster surgical and recovery times. While she opted for a different route, as I said, there is no right answer. Having witnessed this process and standing guard during an extremely intense chemotherapy plan, I personally applaud women who choose this brave option. Whether they are electing this route to reject societal pressures, choosing minimalism/simplicity, or using it as a symbolic gesture (or whatever other reason), I loudly applaud this deeply personal decision. Using this route as a symbolic gesture, perhaps coupled with an "X" tattooed where the nipple previously resided, resonates with people who want to scream "Fuck cancer" from the tallest mountains.

Our long, eventful day at Mayo ended with yet another discussion about nipple-sparing surgery. One more medical advancement that so amazed me. Wendi elected this option, if only to help reduce or cover up scarring. Although the option may not be available at the time of surgery, the doctor concurred with her that it offers a more natural look. And while neither of us could give a shit at the time, he also described that, in some cases, patients can retain sensation in their nipples post-surgery. In these instances, the sensation returns over time. Again, while neither of us could give a damn, I did score this as one more amazing medical advancement.

The Wait Was Almost Over

And with the decision to spare the nipples and reattach, if possible, our long first day at Mayo was complete. We both left numb, exhausted, and uneager to talk on the way home. It was lost on us, at the time, that we never actually discussed whether we would proceed with Mayo as our chosen health provider. During that day, calendars were being set, and our healthcare plan was being created. While not discussed, we were absolutely going forward with Mayo.

Dinner that evening was simple and small, both of us having lost interest in meals ever since receiving the first gut punch. We spent that quiet evening retreating into our own thoughts. Being in full fight-or-flight mode, I thought of all the phone calls I needed to make the next day, thanking those compassionate souls who had offered time/support during our brief yet intense search for both a healthcare team and plan. I also knew I needed to check the box regarding the financial aspects. Although we had very little choice on the matter, I needed to wrap my hands around the out-of-pocket costs and insurance logistics while my energy was still mostly intact. I believe this is crucial at the beginning of the healthcare journey, as financial pressures can feel overwhelming when you are already deeply engaged in the fight, when energy is all but depleted. Getting a handle on the financial aspects of the path ahead helps you place your focus squarely on your loved one during a time when she needs and deserves nothing but your entire attention.

I also noted the need to contact close friends and loved ones, either through a call or text, letting them know of our elected path forward for Wendi's care. We were blessed with a support group that had leaned on each other over the course of so many years. While I suspected they would not fully understand what we were going through, I knew I would occasionally lean on them during our path forward. I also suspected that I would not have the time or energy to push through updates along the way, so I asked one close friend to serve as the conduit for information. I do not do group texts well, so I created a plan to provide our friend with the information to push forward to all.

I vividly remember one more key element after returning home from the Mayo Clinic following our long day of initial meetings. Whether it was spiritual or a result of pure exhaustion (and likely both), I welcomed a profound sense of peace that permeated my very being. The uncertainty and extreme stress that comes with the utter lack of control had dominated our every minute for over two and a half weeks. Faced with so many unanswered questions, coupled with the desperate search for a treatment path and team, fight-or-flight was in pure code red. Every minute.

Before the diagnosis, I felt I had long held on to and developed a good balance in life. A good life comes complete with so many unexpected and unsolicited speed bumps: family challenges, loss of loved ones, societal pressures, financial stress, and loads of other noise and distractions. A good life also comes with many unforeseen moments of happiness and genuine joy. I always viewed joyful moments as life's deposits and stress and turbulence as life's withdrawals. This lovely balance makes a good life complete, providing goosebumps during extreme highs and offering life rafts to navigate extreme lows. I was blessed to have achieved that perspective of balance before receiving gut punch number one, and while nothing could have prepared us for the path ahead, that balance helped bring me peace that evening. Finding Mayo was one of the more important life rafts that the balance of life had ever provided, and that brought me peace that evening. My wife's resolve in making quick decisions brought me peace. And the brief image of a finish line brought me peace.

As I prepared for bed, bathing in that peaceful feeling, I prayed for Wendi's recovery. I prayed for the strength to remain glued to her side. I prayed for our healthcare team, providing her with the experienced care that had been detailed to us. This particular prayer was important, allowing me to let go of the healthcare plan and move it onto the shoulders of the team. Then, I slept. I slept deeply. I slept through an entire evening, for the first time since the first gut punch.

When daylight had already broken, I was groggy but well rested. As my day started, I somehow knew that the peace I had felt the previous evening would not be felt again for a while. I also somehow knew that I would not sleep through an entire night again for a while. What I didn't know was just how long that would be. Days? Weeks? Months? Spoiler alert. As I write this, years following her last treatment, that deep feeling of peace, coupled with a deep sleep through an entire evening, remains elusive to me.

The Weekend Before the Storm

We saw a few close friends that weekend while also beginning our retreat into a state of detachment and isolation. I finished the business side of cancer, which really does suck. With all the stress and uncertainty gripping your every minute, it does not seem right to have this massive economic uncertainty looming like a stress bomb cherry on top. My time was spent understanding deductibles and, more importantly, what would be considered elective under our plan. In direct terms, not covered by insurance.

One bit of happy news, financially, arose. I'm not interested in pushing political ideology, but some bright, compassionate souls in Washington actually came together for some good. My guess is that the Pink Ribbon Brigade, led by ladies with strong convictions, had a hand in this. Irrespective of political beliefs, how breast reconstruction surgery following a mastectomy was treated as elective surgery in the past, and therefore not covered by insurance, is beyond reason. Cancer is definitely nonelective. There is unquestionably a psychological and physical impact associated with a mastectomy. It is unconscionable to think that, prior to the passage of the Women's Health and Cancer Rights Act, many insurance companies treated breast reconstruction following a mastectomy as cosmetic and therefore refused coverage. No longer.

I would love to report that this legislation, correcting a wrong, was approved and celebrated unanimously. Unfortunately, in our broken system, politics were involved. Accordingly, a pure right to correct a wrong like this bill was slid into a broader package of legislation and appropriations. What should have been a stand-alone bill, celebrated by all, was a political tool used to pass through other appropriations. Nonetheless, it passed, and this legislation helped bring awareness and attention to the mastectomy process, bringing stronger insurance coverage for breast cancer patients. Our experience is a testament to this. Starting with our first walk into Mayo, virtually all of the care Wendi received was covered by our policy, making our out-of-pocket expenses mostly limited to meeting deductibles. Bravo to the voices behind the Women's Health and Cancer Rights Act. During a period of extreme stress and uncertainty, no family should face the added burden of financial devastation. Any insurance adjuster who wants to articulate that reconstruction following a mastectomy is cosmetic/elective needs to spend a few moments with the brave ladies involved in the Pink Ribbon Brigade. I am sure these strong ladies would be eager to convince the adjuster otherwise, or perhaps simply offer up an old-fashioned, pink-ribbon ass kicking.

And So It Begins

Following our first of many future Sunday-night scaries, time eventually moved forward, and we drove the twenty-minute trek that Monday morning for our first chemo infusion. Our first treatment day started with an eerie reminder of the COVID lockdown. Before we could enter Mayo and take our place among cancer patients, we had to first endure a drive-thru COVID test in the Mayo parking lot. Given that we were about to spend the day in an infusion room, alongside other cancer patients with low white cell counts, the drive-thru COVID testing made sense. What didn't make sense to me was that Wendi had to endure Nurse Long Stick, each week, very thoroughly swabbing deep into her nose. While Wendi endured Nurse Long Stick, I was only asked questions on the way into Mayo and given a quick temperature check. COVID rarely ever did make sense.

Once her test was deemed clean and my forehead displayed no temp, we were admitted into Mayo. Check-in was almost immediate, and off we went to our first stop, which was a blood draw. Not yet having her chemo port installed, this part looked quite normal. Needle meets arm. Just like that, blood was drawn, and out of Mayo we went, heading to a nearby coffee shop. We didn't know it at the time, but this would become a weekly ritual. Blood was tested weekly to assess cell counts, which helped the healthcare team evaluate vital signs and determine if it would be safe to proceed with chemotherapy. This is a red light/green light process, performed weekly.

The main concern is likely checking the white blood cell count. Chemotherapy weakens the immune system by lowering white cell levels, and the levels can drop drastically, making chemotherapy too dangerous. Close behind white cell count assessment are red cell counts and platelets. Red blood cell counts, if too low, can cause dizziness and shortness of breath, which may necessitate a blood transfusion. Platelets in the system are critical for clotting, and a low platelet count can cause a delay in treatment due to concerns about excessive bleeding. Blood draws also monitor liver and kidney function, as well as evaluate hydration, sodium, potassium, and other factors that could lead to heart irregularities. A lot to watch here for the healthcare team, as they so desperately want to green-light you every week, with an eye toward the finish line.

How do I seem to know so much about the red light/green light process? In this case, it was not from research. I speak from a place of experience, for, as you will soon learn, Wendi was a chemotherapy side-effect unicorn. This was a nickname given to Wendi by her chemo infusion nurse. Throughout our journey, if there was a side effect associated with any of her chemo drugs, it found Wendi. Because of this, the red light/green light process, before treatment, became a massive balancing act. And a source of weekly stress. On one hand, your oncologist wants you to stay on schedule. On the other hand, your healthcare team and caregiver want to keep you safe and ensure that your body will be able to manage the next round of chemo infusion. We came to understand this as treatments progressed, but that first morning, as we sipped coffee and waited for results, we had no reason to think a red light would ever appear.

The Mysterious Infusion Room

Eventually, the call came—it was game on. The first green light was pushed her way, and Wendi's first chemo infusion would happen at noon. This shit was about to get real.

At the time, neither of us knew much about the place known only as *the infusion room.* It carried a kind of mythic weight, a space whispered about in appointments and brochures but rarely explained.

We returned to Mayo and were directed toward an elevator that would take us to the fourth floor. Speaking of four, while we waited longer than usual for an elevator, we noticed a sign limiting each elevator ride to just four people. That meant a patient, a loved one, and a healthcare provider, which left little room for anyone else. Damn COVID. But considering most of the people riding this elevator were likely headed toward the same mysterious room, a little social distancing made perfect sense.

As we waited, I found myself noticing the people around me more than I usually did while in these sterile hospital surroundings. I'm not known for being particularly observant, but this time, the patterns hit me hard. The physical signs of chemotherapy were everywhere. Some had lost their hair entirely. Others wore bright scarves, knit caps, or baseball hats. And some—maybe as a symbolic middle finger gesture to cancer—wore nothing at all, revealing the last wisps of hair without reservation.

Other features also stood out. Some brave souls had lost eyebrows and eyelashes. Most carried a pale, ashen hue, evidence of both the toll of treatment and the isolation of the pandemic. Sunken cheeks, visible weight loss, tired eyes.

And yet . . . their eyes. That's what I'll never forget.

Every one of them had that look—a quiet fire, a gritty kind of focus, like athletes stepping onto the field in the final minutes of a close game. Determined. Resolute. They weren't done fighting. And one thing I knew for sure: No matter how Wendi's appearance might change, she would wear that same fire in her eyes. Quiet determination was her armor.

Speaking of physical appearances, when we reached the fourth-floor waiting area, I leaned over to Wendi and whispered, "Bet you a dollar folks think I am the patient."

She laughed. My beautiful, petite wife of over thirty years had definitely aged much better than I had. My thinning hair and wiry frame didn't help, and on that day, I likely looked more rattled than she did. In truth, she still looked like she could spring from her chair and throw down a roundoff back handspring—a move we occasionally dared her to pull off.

But not on this day.

On this day, we were about to enter a room where people of all ages fought back on a schedule chosen by their oncologists. On this day, we were about to cross a threshold into something that would change us—probably forever, in ways both good and bad.

Watching Wendi as they prepared to call her name, I wasn't worried about the physical changes ahead. Somehow, I knew she had the grit and toughness to weather anything they threw at her. I also somehow knew she wouldn't need me to help her navigate the emotional toll of losing her hair, her eyelashes, or the outer pieces of her identity. Like me, she wouldn't give a damn.

No, if she needed me for anything, it would be to help her see beyond this moment. To believe there was a finish line. That somewhere ahead was a new normal waiting for us—that we could reach one day together.

In a whirlwind of three weeks, we had landed here, standing just steps away from crossing the threshold into the mysterious infusion room.

Wendi, Meet Chemotherapy

Our name was called. And we walked in: one naive, petrified caregiver and one beautiful, strong, courageous mother of four, showing no outward signs of cancer.

The infusion room was massive, stretching across nearly an entire floor of the Mayo Clinic. Its location felt intentional. On the fourth floor in North Scottsdale, its tall windows welcomed Arizona's blue skies and distant mountain ranges. If anyone deserved blue skies and open horizons, it was the souls spending long days tethered to IV poles in this room.

The space resembled a quiet office maze. Cubicles filled much of the room, each containing a large, comfortable reclining chair and a smaller chair with a fold-up tray—just enough space for a loved one to spend the day. Opposite the wall, a series of private glass-walled rooms stood, while nurses' stations and snack areas dotted the rest of the floor.

For a room this size, housing so many people, it was eerily quiet.

That's the strange thing about an infusion room. The emotional weight in the air seems to strike a balance—fear against hope, anxiety against calm. Exhaustion sits opposite resilience, and somehow, those opposing forces coexist in an almost sacred stillness. With so few actual walls—only short distances dividing us—you get the distinct impression that once you're inside, you're part of something collective. You are all in this together. Strength in numbers.

As we followed our nurse on a brief tour, my eyes wandered. Most patients were wrapped in warm blankets, gaining a quiet comfort. Above each recliner, IV poles stood like guards, solemn and constant. Nearly every cubicle held a caregiver or loved one nearby, sitting silently with a book or phone. But every now and then, I saw someone alone. That hit hard. There's something uniquely heartbreaking about fighting this particular battle solo. Bless those brave souls who endure in this manner.

Tour complete, we were led to our first infusion cubicle. And from the moment we sat down, my nerves began to calm—largely thanks to the professionalism and warmth of the care team. After taking Wendi's vitals, two bags of chemo were brought into the cubicle. A second nurse soon appeared. Each bag was carefully labeled and verified against her wristband. One nurse read aloud her name, birth date, and the specific chemo to be administered, while the second nurse double-checked it against the chart.

Precision, clearly, is not optional.

Once verified, the second nurse exited, and the primary nurse walked us through what the day in the infusion room would look like. Because Wendi's chemo port had not yet been installed, they'd start by prepping a vein. Then, they'd begin with a saline flush—essentially a bag of salt water meant to open the vein and clear the lines. The flush, she explained, would help prevent dehydration and serve to reduce chemo side effects. At the time, we simply nodded, grateful for every ounce of explanation.

We didn't know it yet, but that little bag of saline would go on to play a big role in Wendi's treatment days. And while it was supposed to help with hydration, blood pressure, and electrolyte balance, two words would later come to describe it best: no bueno. The hydration bags would become a blessing and a curse, providing her with the fluids she so desperately needed but typically coming once the nasty side effects had done their damage.

Let the Drip Begin

Soon enough, the nurse would begin administering the first two bags of chemotherapy prescribed by our oncologist—drugs to be delivered weekly for twelve consecutive weeks. With her overview complete, precision returned to our cubicle. In short order, Wendi's vein was prepped, the saline was hung, and our hovering IV tower came to life—lit, calibrated, and ready to begin our chemotherapy journey.

Each IV tower in Mayo came equipped with a countdown clock. As a longtime basketball fan, I knew a thing or two about shot clocks and game clocks. But this one was different. Over the course of our treatment calendar, I became fixated on that clock. I watched it like a lifeline—measuring not just time but progress. Every second that passed was one step closer to a finish line.

Beyond the clock, each IV tower emitted a steady beep and low hum. Those sounds became comforting—a quiet white noise that cut through nerves. With the countdown clock set for the saline flush, we listened as the first soft beeps and hums marked the beginning. Drip by drip, Wendi's veins welcomed the first wave. We were off and running.

Strength Comes in Numbers

Oddly enough, my previous fear of hospitals and white coats was never a factor. I was calmed by the presence of others, calmed by the professionalism surrounding us, and calmed by the clarity that comes with action. We were also blessed with an amazing infusion nurse that first day, an individual who approached her newfound role in our lives with positive energy.

Those initial steps into the infusion room felt like the first day of high school—uncertainty, fear, and apprehension all deeply reaching into the soul. With inexperience and uncertainty comes the tendency to conjure up your own monsters. Think back to those books on pregnancy and childcare we all read. Or think back to those Lamaze classes we attended, which tended to be more social than informative and where strength in numbers helped calm fears.

Whether bringing home your first baby, walking into an exam, strolling into a Lamaze class, or stepping into an infusion room, lack of experience breeds uncertainty. With uncertainty comes fear due to the loss of control. If you lose the steering wheel and feel uncertain about the outcome, monsters tend to appear, clouding judgment and bringing anxiety. Major "first-time" experiences breed this uncertainty. But nothing in my past could compare with this.

Looking back, how did we cope with and combat first-time uncertainties? Seems like strength in numbers was always a welcomed friend in those instances. A high school cafeteria, the prep class for an exam, and Lamaze class (a.k.a. social hour) all buoyed our spirits and provided resilience through strength in numbers. In all of those instances, we took solace in having strangers play the role of the naive first-timers alongside us. Together, we rallied, forged new friendships, and shared experiences as we moved forward, slaying uncertainties.

You don't have to look far beyond marriage and children to understand the binding power of shared experience.

Who were your closest friends before you got married? And how about after? If you're like most, you probably felt a subtle gravitational shift toward spending time with other couples. It's not an indictment of earlier friendships—it's simply a testament to the quiet pull of shared experience. The same thing happens when kids enter the picture. And when those kids take up sports, dance, music—whatever path calls them. Before long, your time, conversations, and connections orbit around others walking the same road.

It has nothing to do with the quality of the relationships that came before. Instead, it's about the human need to find comfort, meaning, and strength with those who understand because they're right there too. This is the essence of strength in numbers. It's the steadying comfort of not going through life's hardest chapters alone.

Breast cancer is no exception to this. That's why the Pink Ribbon Brigade is filled with brave souls bound together by a shared reality. And this is likely why so many of them feel called to offer guidance, grace, and strength to those just beginning this journey.

I thought a lot about this as we sat in the infusion room on that first day, my eyes drifting from cubicle to cubicle. All around us were people in various stages of a similar fight, tethered to IV poles, clinging to hope, drawing quiet strength merely from the presence of others who understood.

Strength in numbers. A time-tested, quietly powerful way to face the monsters that lurk in uncertainty—monsters that feed on isolation and inexperience. But when you stand shoulder to shoulder with others, the shadows do tend to shrink.

The Moment Normal Shifted Forever

We eventually settled in with the low hum of the IV tower, accompanied by its steady beep. The countdown clock showed forty-six minutes remaining on that initial saline flush. Quietly, I wished time would slow down, knowing her first chemo infusion was coming up next. But time, indifferent to our pleading, moves on—no matter how fast or slow it feels. Eventually, the clock hit zero, and the IV tower chimed softly, signaling that a bag was empty.

With practiced precision, our infusion nurse appeared, unhooking the bag and tubing with swift efficiency. Into the disposal it went. I suddenly felt lightheaded, holding my breath for what came next. As she described the chemo drugs that would soon enter Wendi's bloodstream—and our lives—my mind reeled. Normalcy was shifting. Instantly. Permanently.

Since the gut punch of the diagnosis, we still had the option, whether we chose it or not, to live as we always had. We could go to dinner, play games, take long walks, and pass time with friends. Despite the looming shadow of cancer, our previous routines remained fully available to us. But now—right here, right now—I understood without needing to be told: That normal was gone. The moment chemo entered her veins, we would cross a threshold we couldn't return from.

It was the difference between having cancer and being treated for cancer. And in that difference lived a subtle kind of grief—the silent goodbye to life as we'd known it. You can't predict how drastically it will change. You just know it will.

As the first bag of chemo was hung on the IV tower, my heart pounded. I had no idea whether this was Taxol or Paraplatin—our oncologist had mapped it all out, but I paid no attention to which one would start the process. I sat frozen, fists clenched, wanting so desperately to stop everything. But the line was hooked up. The timer was set. And without fanfare or ceremony, our normal officially ended. Her chemo had begun.

Wendi's face was unreadable—pure resilience and steel. Mine was anything but. I was a wreck. We didn't say a word, but I know both she and our nurse saw it in my expression. Somehow, over that first countdown—maybe thanks to a calm nurse, a fierce patient, or the rhythmic hum and beep of the IV tower, my panic gave way to a strange, still quiet. I wasn't okay, exactly. But I wasn't unraveling.

In that stillness, my mind had space to drift.

I realized that ever since the gut punch, I'd been in pure fight-or-flight mode—frantically searching for a way forward. That search had consumed every part of me. Between logistics, research, and updates to loved ones, I hadn't considered my next move—what role I'd truly need to play in this fight. That moment was coming.

And it was coming fast.

In Walks a Sentry

As I witnessed the first dose of chemo entering my wife, she calmly slept. The pure exhaustion of the previous weeks was taking over. My mind centered on what was next. At this moment, I knew I could not outwork cancer nor offer any concrete and valued thoughts on her treatment path. I had to relinquish control to the healthcare team, similar to religious faith. I also recognized, as I watched my beautiful wife peacefully sleep, that all control was not lost. I could certainly redirect my energy and exert some control by dedicating my every effort to becoming a pillar at her side, doing whatever was necessary to serve as a loyal caregiver.

This sudden shift in thought and focus was stirred by the dramatic view of watching chemo drugs flow into my loved one's veins. At the time, I was more than naive as to what a caregiver's role was. Love and support, sure. But what else would be required? While I did not understand nor appreciate the role at the time, my mind seemed to avoid the term "caregiver." I found myself searching for a different term, one that captured the energy, strength, and dedication required, while also acknowledging that this role necessitated an emotionless approach. I reached for my phone and searched the term "male caregiver" in the power thesaurus. Unfortunately, up popped things like "male caretaker," "male guardian," and, yes, even "manny." All no bueno. Whenever you see a descriptive term like "manny," time to go rogue. As the countdown clock continued forward, my mind was searching for a descriptive term to describe the role I was about to assume. With the benefit of looking back at our path and journey, I think my mind settled on a fantastic selection that first day.

In walks a sentry. When you envision a sentry, you picture a quiet presence, constantly standing guard. The watchful eye of a sentry brings no additional emotion to an exceedingly emotional journey and depicts the notion of serving as an unyielding, stoic guardian, only engaging in action when called upon. As I shifted my mindset into becoming Wendi's duty-bound sentry, I found myself fulfilling that role, quietly keeping a watchful eye on our surroundings. From the reactions of the healthcare team moving throughout the infusion room to the beeps and hums from the IV tower to the countdown clock, I turned myself into a nonemotional sentry, quietly observing and awaiting to be called into action. Fortunately, on day one, action was limited. Occasionally, she would stir and ask for a blanket, ice chips, or a snack. With any such request, the sentry would spring into action, meeting Wendi's every need before dutifully returning to my post.

First Sighting of the Hazmat Suit

As predicted by the countdown clock, the first bag of chemo eventually ran dry. Our nurse returned to the cubicle, asked Wendi how she was feeling, and calmly confirmed that bag one had been fully deployed into battle. Then, without missing a beat, she began her next routine.

She masked up. A second gown went on. Gloves. A second mask and eye protection. Within seconds, her appearance had transformed. She looked like she was suiting up for a hazardous spill. Suddenly, she appeared as though she was wearing a hazmat suit.

If the naive needed a wake-up call about the potency of chemo drugs, here it was. Watching a professional suddenly dress like she was entering a contaminated zone was all the proof I needed that these drugs were potent and not to be treated lightly. Just as striking was the disposable nature of the gear. Each time she changed bags and tubing, the hazmat suit was shed and discarded. No part of it was reused. The level of care made it clear: What had just entered Wendi's veins was serious business.

Bag two was hung on the IV tower. The tubing was inserted back into Wendi's arm. The countdown clock was reset. And once again, we settled into our positions—Wendi resting quietly and me sinking deeper into my newfound role as her sentry, alert and motionless, ready for any call into action.

But during this round, my internal alarms were screaming.

I couldn't stop scanning her for signs—any hint of a side effect, any flicker of distress. We were new to this, and while I'd read plenty about possible reactions, I had no idea when they would show up—or how. I glanced across the infusion room, watching other patients for clues. Were they reacting? Were they just tired? What was normal?

Minute by minute, the clock moved forward. Eventually, the soft chime of the IV tower signaled that the second bag had nearly run its course. Still no visible side effects. This fresh wave of anxiety proved unnecessary—this time.

Then came the final steps, performed with that same practiced precision. Garments on. Bags removed. Tubes discarded. Garments off. All quickly disposed of.

Chemo Day One was nearly complete.

Our nurse next explained, per our oncologist's orders, that Wendi would receive a strong IV dose of Benadryl—meant to help reduce allergic reactions and inflammation. Once that was administered and the last of the paperwork was handled, we were cleared to leave and fully prepared to walk out.

Well, one of us was.

Wendi tried, briefly, to wave off the wheelchair, but the nurse was having none of it. Wendi was, instead, wheeled out, a sight that would soon become routine in our swiftly evolving normal.

A Brief Chance to Reflect

Following that long first day in the infusion room, Wendi retreated to our bedroom. Her body had just received powerful drugs, and she was physically spent. As she rested comfortably, the house grew quiet—eerily quiet. I wandered through it, suppressing emotions and visuals, continuing my full adjustment into Wendi's steadfast, stoic sentry.

There is a mantra I turn to, in moments like these, when monsters loaded with anxiety start to grow: The past is not as bad as we think, the present not as stressful as it feels, and the future not as uncertain as it can look.

Our minds are masters of magnification, capable of transforming worries into looming disasters. If we loosen the reins too much, the mind becomes a runaway train—plunging into every rabbit hole it can find. Anxiety, when left unchecked, compounds itself. Momentum builds until even the slightest bump can feel like a derailment.

That night, I faced the reality of one of life's greatest fears. Cancer. It had found us. We were now living it. I had to summon every coping strategy I knew of just to stay grounded.

The Past Is Never as Bad as We Imagine

We were married young, right out of college. Not long after our modest honeymoon, graciously funded by an older brother, I told Wendi I wanted to quit my job and apply to law school. Her response was classic Wendi: quick, supportive, and without hesitation.

Looking back, those early years could easily appear overwhelming. I was the first in my family to attend law school, making me naive enough to work my first year. Wendi matched that energy by taking a full-time sales job—and then a second job on weekends and at night.

Three jobs between the two of us while attending law school full-time. Why stop there?

We bought a foreclosed home in Spokane, in a nice neighborhood, but in desperate need of a remodel. Of course we did.

For the first year, we juggled classes, jobs, and endless home improvement projects. I spent days at Gonzaga Law, nights as a grocery store checker, and weekends working on the house. And I had it easy.

Wendi's days started early and ended long after I went to bed. She led the charge on our remodel—stripping wallpaper, painting cabinets, even learning how to install laminate flooring. She did it all.

Sounds like a nightmare, right? Maybe. But only if you let your mind paint it that way.

With distance—and a few glasses of red shared with close friends—those years start to look different. They look formative. Even joyful. In those years, we built a life, learned real skills, found laughter in exhaustion, and left Spokane with a strong marriage and our first baby on the way.

Ask any doctor how medical school and residency felt. Or a football coach about their days as a graduate assistant, living on a couch and working absurd hours. At the time, it all felt like too much. But in hindsight, those early years often become the bedrock of who we are.

Perspective shrinks monsters. The past just wasn't all that bad.

The Present Is Not as Stressful as We Can Make It

The present, on the other hand, is trickier—because we're living in it. Every red light, every unreasonable client, every surprise bill in the mail can feel like a trigger. Normal life is full of noise, and anxiety prospers best in noise.

But life gives us tools.

Movement. A walk, a run, yoga—any form of exercise. Movement produces endorphins, clears the fog, and slows the runaway train. Even stillness can be a tool. Meditation, breathwork, a good book, a podcast, a favorite TV show.

Which tool is best? The one that works for you. Once you find it, own it. Make it a habit. Habits change narratives, and new narratives can shrink monsters.

The storm we feel isn't always the storm that is.

The Future Is Never as Uncertain as It Looks

And then there's the future—the blank canvas, the unpainted page. When left unchecked, our minds can paint what they want, which is typically a horror story.

Our minds thrive when free to write worst-case scenarios. We fill in shadows that have yet to be formed, only to allow anxiety to grow. We imagine losses we haven't faced and grief that hasn't arrived. That sort of anxious projection, creating worst-case scenarios, paralyzes us.

But there are ways to rein this in.

By softening the narrative of the past and properly grounding ourselves in the present, we narrow the range of the future. The stories we tell ourselves become more measured, more accurate. The future will still bring surprises, both beautiful and painful, but they won't hit quite as hard. The edges won't feel as sharp. The shadows won't seem as deep.

That quiet, sleepless night, I summoned every tool I had. Cancer was no longer a distant fear hiding in the closet next to a monster. It had stepped fully into the room. Into the daylight. And with it came a new kind of silence—heavy, humbling, and unavoidable.

So I landed on tools that long evening to help me manage through our journey ahead. I circled dates on the calendar. Weddings. Trips we wanted to take. Concerts. Anything we could look forward to, so vitally important now. Anchors in the storm. Visual proof that there was still a future worth chasing.

And I remembered one more tool—something I call a "parlor trick." It runs contrary to our deepest instincts, especially in crisis. It's simply this: Try loosening your grip.

Let me explain.

Our minds crave control. When we feel powerless, we grip tighter. We look for guarantees. But that grip can generate more anxiety than relief, particularly when things do not go as planned. What if, instead, we applied light pressure? What if we practiced letting go, if just a little?

Think of a self-driving Tesla. You enter your destination, and the car handles most of the journey—speed, navigation, even lane changes and signals. It asks but one thing of you, as the driver: Keep a light grip on the wheel. Let go entirely, and the self-driving feature shuts off. Over-grip the wheel, and the car won't turn easily. But keep a steady, gentle hand on the wheel, and it lets you go where you need to go.

The same can be true of navigating fear.

Light pressure. Not control, not surrender. Just presence. And a little dash of faith.

That night, in the dark, I landed in a place of strange clarity. The past didn't seem so bad. Present-day stressors shrank into irrelevance. And the future?

Let's be honest. One of the biggest monsters the mind can conjure up is cancer, in any form. And now that monster wasn't lurking in a closet—it was real. It had moved in, taken a seat at our table, and made itself at home.

In doing so, it pushed all the other monsters aside.

Winds Slowing, For Now

As my mind wandered through ways to cope with our quickly evolving normal, Wendi rested. Food held little interest for her, nor did conversation or television. She and her now very clingy poocher retreated to our bedroom, the dog not leaving her side as she rested and scrolled on her phone. Other than making sure her Yeti was constantly filled with water, I wasn't called upon much that first evening following her initial treatment.

She wasn't showing any side effects yet, but the ever-dutiful sentry remained on high alert, ready to leap into action. I'd done the research and asked all the probing questions I could. I had no practical experience managing side effects, but I was ready to react the moment she showed any sign. For now, Wendi and her loyal pooch, Winter, breathed rhythmically, resting peacefully.

Before treatment began, I'd appointed a dear friend to serve as the point person—to share information I passed along with other loved ones. We utilized this hub-and-spoke approach to communication: I'd tell one, and she would inform the others. It worked quite well as treatments progressed and energy waned.

Most of my other communication that night was with our kids, especially my second-oldest daughter. Cassandra Mary had always been the protective type—Mama Bear mode came naturally to her. During this process, she stepped up big, keeping watch over both her mom and me whenever she could. I wish she hadn't had to witness the more brutal parts of treatment, but I cannot imagine how we would've made it through without her.

Guardian Angels Do Exist

I started a Monday-night ritual: walking laps between the living room and bedroom, scanning for any shiver of movement that might require action. I also had a phone call to make, something I was still building the strength for. But I didn't want to stray too far from my post. The sentry doesn't wander. Looking back, it is truly astounding how naive and inexperienced I was following the first treatment. I was rolling on adrenaline and stoic concentration, devoid of any knowledge or training. Thank God for guardian angels.

There was a gent in my life who, after learning of Wendi's diagnosis, opened up about his own gut punch. Over a decade earlier, he and his wife had begun their own fight—for their beautiful daughter. He had spent long nights in hospitals, and through sheer necessity and curiosity, he learned a lot about chemo and, unfortunately, side effects. When Wendi's treatment plan was outlined, he tried to educate me. But early on, the terms he used meant little to me. The side effects he described felt abstract, like something from another planet. I felt confident that this could not happen to us.

As Wendi's journey progressed, he became my confidant. My guardian angel. He had a knack for showing up when I needed him most. And while the male gene might block many of us from sharing openly, in a time of crisis, I can't recommend enough finding someone who's been there—someone who can do more than just listen. Someone, instead, who gets it.

I've never been good at asking for or accepting help. But he offered his number and insisted I use it. He probably regretted that offer at times, but for the next eight months, he stayed on my speed dial. He was one of the few people I could talk to who truly understood what the hell was happening. Much like the fierce Pink Ribbon Brigade who circle around newly diagnosed sisters, he paid it forward—offering strength, insight, and hope that, yes, we could make it through this.

Not to generalize—maybe to observe—but women tend to share feelings more freely than men. That is a true gift, which certainly helps to unpack emotions. Unfortunately, I, like most of my close friends, do not have this gift, and we tend to keep these feelings to ourselves. Before the gut punch came, I internalized everything. Rarely cried. Kept emotions bottled up. But once I stepped into the role of sentry, emotional isolation became an absolute necessity. I saw myself as a flight attendant during heavy turbulence—passengers looking for reactions to calm anxiety. I believed Wendi, our kids, our friends, and our loved ones would all be looking to me in much the same way. So I stayed calm. I kept still. I broadcasted strength, regardless of how I was feeling.

But with my guardian angel, I didn't need to do any of that. He already knew and would read right through it. With him, I could let my guard down, shift out of sentry mode, and talk to him as Paul, not Sentry Paul.

With Wendi resting, I made the first of many calls to him. He picked up immediately, seemingly expecting the call. Just by picking up, he fulfilled his promise and showed me that he would be there for me. He fired off questions—about treatment, how she was responding. His grasp of the details was remarkable, and his tone gave me comfort. He wasn't clinical like the nurses had been—he spoke like someone who'd lived it. I moved easily into full sponge mode, soaking up his wisdom and his watch-out list, making mental notes I'd reference more often than I cared to admit. His consistent approach throughout the process, besides just listening, was to arm me with information and tools, just in case.

Spoiler alert: "Just in case" happened almost every time.

The Dreaded Side Effects Better Understood

I knew my guardian angel was always hoping for the best—but I think he also saw Wendi's petite frame and somehow knew what might be coming. He tried to prepare me, gently arming me with a list of what to watch out for. For Wendi's specific chemo cocktail, here were the big potential side effects he described:

Fatigue. Not the kind of tired you can fix with a nap. This was gravity-altering exhaustion—like Earth had tilted and was now pulling her down harder. It's a fatigue that apparently flips your body upside down, inside out, and refuses to let go.

Nausea, vomiting, and metallic taste. Nausea made sense—powerful drugs were invading her system. Nausea seems like a likely result. But the metallic taste was something I hadn't expected. It made food unappealing, which would only make the nausea worse, especially when vomiting entered the picture. Battling nausea on an empty stomach is simply not a fair fight.

Dehydration. The dirty "D." Staying properly hydrated can become quite a chore. Add nausea, vomiting, metallic taste, and extreme fatigue to the mix, and suddenly even sitting up to sip water can feel like a mountain climb. Everything can appear to conspire to steal fluids—quickly. And disappearing fluids bring the dirty "D" into the picture, front and center.

Neuropathy. A new word for me. Tingling, numbing sensations in the fingers and toes—what Wendi would later describe as static electricity dancing just beneath her skin.

Body aches. These were described as flu-like soreness, intensified by inactivity and vomiting. A body, already undergoing chemical warfare, would be crying out from the sudden shift in routine and the internal chaos happening as a result of the chemo cocktail.

Fever. My guardian angel stressed this one. And highlighted it constantly. "Buy digital thermometers," he said. "And lots of them." And I did. The no-touch kind was especially helpful—I could take her temperature without waking her and, lots of times, without her noticing I was stealing this information from her body. Looking back after the fact, I won't even guess how many times I tiptoed into the bedroom to steal a temp check. Our wood floors were a blessing—had it been carpet, it would've shown a well-worn path straight to her forehead.

Rigors. Saved the worst for last. Chemotherapy was already the "C word" in my vocabulary, a word I could not (or would not) say out loud. Rigors soon became yet another forbidden term, stricken from my vocabulary out of self-preservation. I had to look it up again, years later, just to be sure I remembered it correctly. I had buried it that deep.

Rigors are violent, uncontrollable chills. Think of being caught outside in a snowstorm for a week. You finally find shelter, wrap yourself in blankets, but your body won't stop shaking. Your teeth chatter. Your muscles seize. Now multiply that thought by five. Or ten. That's the way rigors were described. Blankets don't help. Medication barely touches it. Even love—deep, unflinching love—can't soothe it.

Rigors is a nasty, unrelenting bitch. And she's immune to everything but time.

Maybe We Are the Lucky Ones

After soaking in every warning about side effects—from research, the medical team, the Pink Ribbon Brigade, and my guardian angel—you can certainly understand why I didn't sleep that first night. Or, really, any night.

But she slept. Peacefully, even. And when morning came after the day of her first infusion, she woke up tired but *hungry*. Maybe "hungry" is a bit of a stretch, but it was the first time she'd asked for food since the gut punch had arrived. After a small meal, she even began planning out the day—a walk, later, if the weather held.

For a moment, this stoic sentry almost let his guard down. Hope crept in—dangerous, seductive hope. Maybe, just maybe, we were among the lucky ones. The ones who would slip through the cracks of probability, untouched by the worst of it. Maybe, just maybe, her body would not react to the chemicals in a manner that would take her to her knees. On that warm spring day, there was no way to know how short-lived that hope would be. No way to know the storm that lay ahead—ferocious, unrelenting, and unlike anything we could've imagined.

The rest of that first posttreatment week gave us reason to be cautiously optimistic. Wendi was up and moving about, showing no major side effects beyond fatigue. Our daughter Cassey was visiting from Boise, which gave Wendi a much-needed lift. She even planned a few small social outings with close friends—an effort, I think, to hold on to the last strands of our fading normal. Likely designed for me more than her.

Most impressively, she suggested a hike. Not a walk, but a real hike. An 1,100-foot climb to watch the sunrise. Her idea. And we did it. There were moments she looked ready to turn back, but every time, she found the will to push forward, summoning strength from somewhere deep within her. Against the odds, we made it to the top and stood together, gazing over Scottsdale as the sun rose that morning. I remember looking around at the faces and the scenery below, not wanting that moment to end.

That evening, after a quiet dinner on the patio with Cassey, Wendi made an unexpected announcement: She wanted to face the hair inevitability—on her own terms.

I wasn't ready. Not even close to ready. But Cassey, who'd inherited more than just Wendi's strength (strength can surely be substituted with stubbornness in this context), sprang immediately into action. Before I could express an opinion or object, they were both laughing and crying as Cassey buzzed away the hair. I stayed quiet, locked in early sentry mode, watching this transformation unfold with my emotions packed in tightly, buried deep.

Seeing her hair scattered across the patio floor was a quiet gut punch of its own. I swept it up silently, knowing the moment on that mountaintop might've been the last time I was fully myself—not hidden behind the armor of the ever-watchful sentry.

I never researched this part—this emotional retreat, this mental discipline of the stoic sentry. I saw this as necessary. I researched her journey and made mental notes of the various side effects that could be potentially experienced along the way. If I missed even one detail, one symptom, one change in her physical condition, I might fail her. I simply believed that I couldn't let that happen. I couldn't let her down. And so, I could not afford to feel overwhelmed. Or sad. Or, really, anything. This led me to the conclusion that, for her sake, I had to bury the emotions. Deep. And bury the shovel behind them.

Watching my daughter shear away the last bits of Wendi's hair was my first true test of emotional isolation. And I passed. On the outside. Inside, it cut deep—but I kept it there, inside, where it wouldn't interfere. I had a job to do and a role to play. The job was to stay vigilant. Stay focused. The role was to appear strong at all times. And quietly sweep up the remnants of normal as they fell to the ground.

And the Sunday Scaries Intensify

As the sun officially set on what had been a surprisingly peaceful week, the Sunday scaries crept back in. Monday meant treatment number two—and Sunday night, in our new normal, became a portal to dread.

Back in our old life, our previous normal, the Sunday scaries were mostly mild. Just the mental shift from weekend ease to workweek pace and stress. But now, in this shifting normal, they arrived like another punch to the gut. This wasn't about meeting a deadline or presenting to a client—this was chemo. This shit was now so very real. And even though week one had gone better than expected, the uncertainty of what lay ahead had us both wide-eyed in bed, staring into the dark ceiling above.

We tossed. We turned. We tried to pretend it wasn't coming. We both knew sleep would help with the days ahead, but the anxiety made sleep unreachable. And for me—as the sentry—sleep aids simply were not an option. I needed to be sharp, ready, alert. I knew her next wave of side effects could be around any corner. And so the night dragged on, my mind barricaded against much-needed rest by fear and what-ifs.

Checking the time only made it worse. It always does. Each glance at the clock felt like a countdown to battle. We were now just hours from the twenty-minute drive back to Mayo.

Then Wendi broke the silence. "You need some sleep."

Captain Obvious, sure—but it still touched me that she was thinking of me in that moment. She turned on her side, and soon her breathing evened out. That soft rhythm—so familiar, so human, so Wendi—had a calming effect. Slowly, panic and anxiety began to loosen their grips. The Sunday scaries, fierce as they were, began to retreat. And with it, the no-sleep dragons were slain.

Of course, sufficient sleep or not, Monday still came. I jumped out of bed with the alarm, trying to fake some appearance of control. I convinced Wendi to eat a light breakfast and doubled down on her fluids. Her prep time to leave the house had shrunk considerably. Comfortable sweats. A knit cap. Makeup now a relic from our previous normal. A different life. Her ever-loyal poocher sensed something was off again—circling the door, barking incessantly as we left the house.

Round Number Two

I tried to make small talk on the drive to Mayo, but small talk was going the way of makeup—fading quickly. Our nerves were quietly firing off, but I stayed in full sentry mode, burying emotion deep, summoning calm where there was none.

We moved through the familiar pretreatment gauntlet: COVID drive-thru (yes, with Nurse Long Stick)—check. Temperature screen—check. Blood draw—check. Wait at the nearby coffee shop for the green light to the infusion room via Mayo's incredible app—check.

It's rather amazing how fast you can adapt to a completely new routine that, just weeks ago, didn't exist.

Around noon, the app gave us the go-ahead. The hope for the green light landed positively, and soon I was wheeling a much different-looking Wendi into the infusion room. It was slowly becoming obvious which of us was the patient. We skipped the tour of the infusion room this time and were directed straight to our treatment cubicle. I looked at her and said, "Only fifteen to go." Over time, this became our little ritual—a quiet acknowledgment that there was, in fact, a finish line somewhere ahead, irrespective of whether we could see it.

This was her last infusion without a chemo port. Same drugs, same drip, same sounds emitting from the IV tower. But none of these familiarities made it any easier.

I sat in sentry posture—offering snacks, liquids, blankets, anything in my arsenal. Wendi slept through both infusions that day. As she rested, I used the time to question our nurse, trying to understand what exactly was being pushed into my wife's veins.

The gut punch was still recent, and I was still playing catch-up on the terminology and the process. I admitted to the nurse that this all felt like poison to me. She didn't dismiss this thought. These were cytotoxic drugs—"toxic" right there in the name. Their job was to kill cells. All of them. Cancerous, yes—but healthy ones too.

That thought messed with my mind quite a bit. How do you reconcile poison as medicine? These chemicals didn't discriminate. They weren't gentle. They were not kind. They were necessary, yes, but brutal. Intense. And yet the nurses, the entire infusion team, delivered these brutal, toxic drugs with such compassion, carrying with them the internal conviction that the pain these drugs were inflicting had a purpose.

I needed that reminder. I needed to believe in the logic of this treatment, even when everything in me wanted to rip the IV out and run. Over time, that internal tug-of-war only grew more intense. Watching the effects take hold, over time, made me hate those chemo drugs, irrespective of their long-term purpose. But on that day, that second day of treatment, as I sat dutifully beside her, I accepted the paradox: Each treatment was both harm and hope. Poison in exchange for time. Damage, traded for the chance at more days together.

The compassion of the healthcare team helped me hold onto that fragile balance. My role remained clear: Remain steady while the medicine and the people administering the medicine waged their war. Sentries don't question. Sentries don't blink.

Even Distant Finish Lines Can Be Seen

As infusion number two slowly dripped into Wendi's veins, I realized I needed something more. Something to hold onto. Fourteen more treatments lay ahead of this day, which seemed like such a heavy weight, an almost insurmountable challenge. Given this knowledge, I felt the need to have a vision—something to help make sense of the road ahead of us. A visual to grasp and help my conviction and commitment to this process.

I'm a visual person. Always have been. I needed a finish line I could see in my mind, something that helped give meaning to the brutal calendar we were now living by. I also have always viewed finish lines as something that held much more meaning when not crossed alone.

The image that I so desperately wanted came to me with almost no effort. It had already been living quietly in my heart.

While living in Barcelona, my oldest daughter and son-in-law gave us one of life's most beautiful gifts: our first grandbaby, Olivia. From the moment she arrived, she absolutely owned us. Because of the distance between us, our time with Olivia came in precious, compact doses. But when we were together, we were all in. Fully present. Fully smitten. This little bundle of joy captured our everything.

So, as Wendi rested beside me and the chemo continued to wage its slow, quiet war, I began to visualize a future. Our future. A real, tangible future. Beach days. School recitals. Soccer games. Time on the lake. All of it with Olivia. And, most importantly, all of it with Wendi there, holding Olivia's hand, cheering her on, making memories.

These mental images became sacred. It was the thing I clutched onto during the darkest moments ahead, the thing I replayed when fear began to build stories I didn't want to read. That visual—so simple, so powerful—reminded me that we had the power to write our own ending. The outcome wasn't fixed. Not yet.

I must've replayed these scenes hundreds of times throughout our journey. Each time Wendi faced yet another side effect, another setback, I would close my eyes and go there. To our visualized future. To the beach. To the recital hall. To the sidelines of a soccer match. If only for a second, those images pulled me forward, helped me imagine life beyond the war zone.

That vision of Olivia and the future she represented didn't erase the pain. It didn't boost energy. But it gave the pain purpose, and it offered reassurance when energy levels dwindled. It provided internal strength to a sentry. And these visions reminded me of one important, nay vital, fact in life. Even the most distant finish lines can be seen if you're willing to keep looking.

Wishing Side Effects Were Merely Warning Labels

After two chemo bags, a saline flush, and a dose of antihistamine were delivered, our second day in the infusion room was in the books. More than five-plus hours in our cubicle, and we thought we were getting a handle on things. But that feeling didn't last very long at all.

During the twenty-minute drive home from Mayo, I started noticing signs. She'd slept most of the day during treatment, but her exhaustion now felt deeper. Her color was off—pale, with shadows forming under her eyes. Something had shifted.

When we got home, she skipped food and headed straight for bed, her ever-faithful poocher close behind, happy to have Wendi back home. I followed soon behind with crackers, electrolyte water, and a list of gently asked questions. I also took her temperature. It wasn't alarming—yet—but it was already a little high.

She let me layer down the blankets and sipped a bit of water before closing her eyes, exhaustion creeping in. I turned the TV on for background noise, more for me than her, and resumed my watch. I was officially back on patrol—marching between the living room and the bedroom, listening for breathing patterns, checking her temperature, scanning her body language for anything potentially off.

We'd arrived home just before 6 p.m. By 9:30, I'd already done eight to ten temp checks, quietly fighting off rising alarms within my head. Something wasn't right. But this was instinct talking, not experience.

Then I heard her stir. I walked in with the thermometer in hand, and there she was: pale, shivering, quietly crying. She said her skin was tingling, her body cramping. She asked for another blanket.

I took her temp—now officially in the triple digits. She was cold, so cold—but burning up. And just like that, the unicorn of side effects had arrived.

That's what we came to call it. The full-on, no-holds-barred combo of chemo side effects. The worst of the worst. Rigors were now fully in our bedroom, impersonating my wife, and our new normal had taken a violent turn neither of us had seen coming.

Armed with no experience, no tools, and no formal training, I moved into action. Cold washcloth on the forehead. More water in the Yeti. Soft encouragement to help her avoid the extra blanket. All of these on-the-fly moves felt like flu care—simple moves used with kids, which showcased my lack of training and tools. While I performed these simple tasks, I wasn't naive. I knew better. This wasn't the flu. This was war.

And I was outmatched.

The cold compress helped. She also finally agreed to sit up, sip some water, and nibble on a cracker. I took a moment of relative calm to call Mayo's after-hours oncology line for the first time—a number that would become memorized and deeply worn into my call history over the months ahead.

The nurse answered, pulled up Wendi's chart, and calmly asked some questions. She wanted to better understand how this Monday night differed from last Monday. After gathering the details, she promised to call back—and she did. Promptly. She'd reached our oncologist. Just like that, two prescriptions were approved: one for nausea, the other to help with pain from rigors.

And there it was—that word again. Rigors. A word I had attempted to bury, suddenly dug up now like a bad memory with claws.

She told me to give Wendi Tylenol but to monitor use closely. They didn't want me to overly mask the fever—merely attempt to best manage it. She encouraged me to call back if things escalated. And with the prescriptions and instructions for monitoring fever spikes being pushed out, she hung up. The line went quiet. And I held the phone for a moment, realizing that, once again, the sentry was alone.

I couldn't leave Wendi to pick up the prescriptions, so I went back to my post, with no additional ammo to rely upon. Tylenol. Fresh compress. More water. More broken-record pleading for her to drink additional fluids. And more temp checks. I had a mental redline—102 degrees—at which point I was told to call back immediately by the nurse. While we never reached it that evening, the margin was razor-thin.

Her temp eventually dropped a bit. The aches, pains, and chills softened. She found her way to some shallow sleep. I stayed close, waking her regularly for sips of water, the thermometer in constant rotation. And as I sat there, watching her breathe, I realized again, this wasn't anything like caring for a sick child with the flu. There were certainly similarities—washcloths, fluids, endless worry—but the stakes were unimaginably higher. And the pressure was much more intense.

With chemo, every upward tick in temperature is a potential emergency. Every cramp or tremble could mean something more. These aren't just symptoms; they're signals. These are things that can delay treatment. They can threaten progress. They can turn everything sideways in a heartbeat.

That night, I sat in a chair pulled up beside her bed and stared into the darkness. No books. No distractions. Just the shallow rhythm of her breath and the weight of what I didn't know. Outside, the world spun like any normal evening. But inside our house, I felt completely, profoundly alone.

I won't call it despair. I still won't. But it was heavy, like a trench you don't know how to climb out of. The responsibility. The lack of experience. The isolation. It all met at the same intersection that night. And though the worst side effects were still to come in the weeks ahead, that sleepless Monday night was the hardest for me. It was the first full test—of strength, faith, endurance.

Normal Doesn't Change for Everyone in Unison

That long, sleepless night revealed something I hadn't fully processed until then: We were in this alone. Not because people didn't care—God, they did. We were blessed with loving, compassionate friends and loved ones. But their normal hadn't been uprooted like ours. Their normal was no longer within the same zip code.

Wendi was on their minds. I knew that. They checked in, sent meals, and offered help. But they still went to work, attended social events, lived their lives. As they absolutely should. Their world hadn't shifted—while ours had cracked wide open. Almost immediately following the gut punch, our lives were following completely different trajectories.

And there's no blame in that. Truly. Just because our normal changed so suddenly and so dramatically didn't mean theirs had to. Life doesn't freeze for everyone just because your world stops spinning. That's not selfish. It's just another reality that follows a gut punch.

Still, I couldn't help but feel the distance growing. Not in the typical manner, like having some fear of missing out. No, this was much different. Priorities had changed, and the concept of FOMO was nonexistent. Once, we'd all walked the same roads—careers, marriages, kids. We celebrated together, struggled through growing pains side by side. But now, suddenly, our ship had veered off course. The storm had hit us alone, pulling us away from our pack. They couldn't possibly understand what we were facing—not fully. And in some strange way, I didn't want them to.

I didn't want to pull them into this. I didn't want them to feel the heaviness of it. My "pleaser" gene, forged by a childhood of moving around and trying to fit in, kicked into overdrive. I felt an almost compulsive need to protect our loved ones from the raw truth of our new normal. Not just to spare them, but maybe to spare us. Retelling it, reliving it, unpacking the emotions and the details? That would only drain us more and perhaps stall our burning desire to keep pushing forward. After all, reliving this new reality through unpacking details could risk causing more pain and less progress.

Right or wrong, I made a quiet decision. I'd keep them informed, but only at a distance. High-level updates. Nothing too deep. Nothing that would pull them into the dark. Our dark. Yes, this would cause further isolation and force me to bury the imagery and emotions of our new normal. But isolation felt like the safer choice. It was better to keep others at a distance than pull them into the trenches with us.

By then, only two weeks into treatment, I already understood: You can't truly comprehend this new normal—our new normal—unless you're living it. And I wouldn't wish that kind of knowledge or understanding on anyone.

So I created a shield, around them and around us. Let them keep their normal. Let them stay warm on much calmer seas. I'd face the wind. Whatever storms brewed ahead, I would navigate alone with Wendi.

So much for strength in numbers. Damn that gut punch.

Daylight Comes and I Want to Go Home

Eventually, that long Monday evening passed. As sunlight broke through the windows, the monsters retreated into their corners—for a while, at least.

Because I never fell asleep, there was no immediate hope upon seeing the sunlight that I was concluding a bad dream. No, this wasn't a bad dream. There was no moment of waking relief. The gut punch was as real as it gets, and daylight only confirmed it.

Wendi wasn't back to herself that morning, but she was much calmer. Her fever had broken. She was more cooperative with fluids—and less inclined to swear at the sentry when he denied her a blanket. Let's call that progress.

I stayed with her through the morning, watching, monitoring, waiting. When I finally felt comfortable enough to step away, I threw on a hat and made the pharmacy run to pick up the meds prescribed the night before.

On the way, I called my guardian angel. I needed to talk. I can't overstate what it meant to have someone on the other end of the line who already knew—someone who didn't need me to explain the difference between fear and panic, between tired and depleted. He got it. All of it.

I described Wendi's side effects in detail. He offered insights, validation, and suggestions. But more than that, he listened. Fully. Patiently. Like someone who had lived it and was willing to live it again—for my sake. Such a sacrifice, but perhaps another form of unpacking was happening right before my eyes that I didn't recognize at the time?

That call gave me more than just advice. It gave me breath. Energy. Perspective. And a reminder: I wasn't entirely alone. Not with him on the other end of the line.

When I got home, Wendi was curled up on the bed, completely drained. The fever was gone, but it had taken her energy with it. She showed no interest in food and barely left the bedroom for days.

And yet, even in that state, Wendi held tight to scraps of our previous normal. Later that week, after moving from the bedroom to the living room, she announced she'd made dinner plans with close friends. On Saturday. Five days post-infusion. After rigors.

After a burning fever. After a complete system crash. And yet, for her, something to look forward to.

Everything in me wanted to push back. But that's not what sentries do. We don't veto. We support. We watch. We honor. We love. And so, what Wendi wanted, Wendi would get. A Saturday night with friends it will be, reluctance be damned.

A Haircut for a Sentry

If Wendi was going out Saturday night, I felt I needed to make one change of my own. She was losing her hair, at least the remaining strands that Cassey didn't clip in the makeshift, backyard barber shop. These remaining strands of hair she would lose on her own terms. I didn't see any reason she should be the only hairless one in the household. Especially not if she was going to venture out into public.

So, while she rested on the couch, I slipped out for an hour and headed to my Russian barber. As I climbed into the chair, I told him we were going for a different look. A hard reset.

When he eventually heard the reason for this change, he didn't hesitate. He moved the clippers to their shortest setting and went to work. In absolutely no time, I was hairless. Fully committed. As I stood to pay, avoiding the mirror for the moment, he waved me off—forcefully—and offered a heartfelt wish for Wendi's recovery. He also offered to help clean up her scalp anytime she needed. There's real compassion in our world. Generosity does not have to come in large buckets. I'll never forget his simple, kind gesture.

Back home, I'm not sure Wendi was thrilled about the new look. In hindsight, I think it felt like a constant reminder of our new normal, looking at this shift in my appearance. For me, though, it was a no-brainer. On our first trip to the infusion room, Wendi still looked like her old self—cheerful, healthy. There was confusion in people's eyes over who the actual patient was. As a way of protecting her, I wanted that confusion to continue. If we were going out, I wanted eyes on me—not on her.

Before Saturday night arrived, another change to our routine was scheduled. Friday was port infusion day—no more IV sticks in the arm. No more blood draws with needles. No more bruises. No more visible reminders that made her flinch every time.

The procedure was fast. In and out in about forty minutes. She came out a bit groggy but calm. It was a small medical step forward but a big emotional one. The port meant quicker access for blood draws and chemo infusions, offering her less trauma, less stress. But it was also another mark—one more sign that normal had shifted.

The port itself created a subtle bump under the skin, just below the collarbone. The Pink Ribbon Brigade had warned her: some tops, most bras, and some dresses would no longer be practical. Certain fabrics would irritate it. She would need to lean into soft, loose-fitting clothes as her new go-to. Fashion statements be damned. These were small changes, but like the rest, they added up. Quiet losses. Small farewells to the life we once knew.

A Not-So-Simple Night Out

By Saturday evening, Wendi looked rested and determined. We had both a daughter and our son in town, and we were joining close friends for dinner—our first real night out since the gut punch arrived. Our daughter, the resident foodie, picked a spot in downtown Phoenix we had not tried before. Against the sentry's better judgment, we loaded into the car and went searching for something that resembled our old normal.

We must've been quite a sight—Wendi in a loose-fitting dress and knit cap, me freshly bald. But we were committed. We were doing it. We were out.

We filled a large table—three families that, over the years, had blended into one. For a brief moment, it felt . . . real. I even ordered my first cocktail following her diagnosis. Banter flowed. Laughter felt effortless. For the first time in well over a month, I allowed myself to exhale.

As is so typical, Wendi had been right. We needed this.

What I didn't realize until that very moment, sitting there with a drink in hand and conversation swirling around us, was that this night wasn't for her—it was for me. She'd planned it, pushed for it, insisted on it . . . for me. Even as she carried the weight of chemo treatment, even as her body betrayed her, she was thinking of me and my well-being.

And just as I let my guard down and took my armor off, just as I stepped out of sentry mode for the first time since the beginning of chemo treatment, our new reality came crashing in.

No warning. No sign. One moment, she was upright, laughing softly. The next, she slumped forward—eyes rolled back, body going limp. The restaurant seemed to freeze. Time stood still. My son, sitting across from her, looked over at me with wide, terrified eyes.

I snapped back into sentry mode instantly. Cold compress. Knit cap off. Our daughter was already at Wendi's side, holding her upright, calling her name. Friends at the table jumped in without hesitation, one of them helping to form a plan while I sprinted to get the car, air-conditioning blasting.

By the time I pulled up, the friend who formed the plan was carrying Wendi through the restaurant, every pair of eyes tracking them like a spotlight. He delivered her gently into the front seat, and we drove off—our daughter in the back seat, our son left behind in stunned silence.

For a moment, I didn't know where we were headed. Home? Or Mayo? But with the cold air on her face and her color returning, Wendi came back. Slowly. The answer was that we were going to head home.

Once she was settled and resting, I stayed up late with my son. A college athlete, he'd been mostly away. This was the first time he'd seen his mom since her treatment began. What he saw that night, what none of us expected, ripped the veil off everything for him. He was abruptly welcomed into our new normal.

Basketball—the game he loved, lived, and breathed—suddenly meant less. That night, it became what it was: just a game.

He was shaken. Scared. Desperate for reassurance. He wanted to leave school. Quit the team. Come home. Be close.

I couldn't give him what he really wanted. What he so desperately needed. I couldn't say, "Everything's going to be okay." I couldn't say it because I didn't know if that was true. So, instead, I told him what I did know. Mom was the strongest person in our family. She was getting the best care possible. We had a support system. It was our turn to lift her up.

As we talked deep into the night, I saw something shift in him. A quiet transformation. I spoke openly about her diagnosis, the treatment plan, and the possible reasons behind what happened at dinner that night. He listened, wide-eyed, fixed on me like a passenger watching a flight attendant during heavy turbulence.

And I played my role. Calm. Measured. No false promises. Just the facts surrounding our new normal and the strength I could offer.

That night, my son took a rather large step toward manhood, progress likely delayed a bit due to COVID. He felt the weight of our new normal. He saw his mother in her most vulnerable state. And he chose to stand beside her. Although he ultimately made the right decision to return to school, he was willing to give it up. In his mind, within this new normal, basketball could wait. Life—real life—had taken the court.

Sunday: No Longer the Fun Day

The Sunday after Wendi's big night out started quietly. A light family walk, mostly through the neighborhood. A small, simple dinner. It almost felt like a gentle reset. But, of course, it didn't last.

That night, as we climbed into bed, the Sunday scaries returned—amplified now by everything we'd experienced the week before, along with the fainting episode that was still fresh in our minds. Sleep didn't stand a chance. The tossing and turning started early. Our bodies were exhausted, but our minds were hijacked by "what-ifs."

In our previous normal, our old lives, Sundays meant the end of leisure and the start of a workweek. A little stress, a little sighing, nothing too serious, regardless of how it felt at that moment. But now, Sundays were a warning siren. The eve of battle. And each one carried the weight of knowing what Monday would bring: more chemicals, more side effects, more unknowns.

The mind is a cruel narrator during these nights. It invents scenes. Replays worst-case scenarios. Magnifies shadows until they become monsters. And no matter how illogical those thoughts are, they build a barricade between you and rest.

Each time I checked the clock, I felt the pressure mount. Time crawled. The drive to Mayo loomed in the morning ahead.

During our drive to Mayo for treatment number three, I noticed her complexion had faded further. Her shoulders were starting to slump. That strong, athletic frame now seemed carved down to essentials: bone, skin, and the will to fight.

The saline flush started the day. The bags of chemo soon followed, dripping slowly. And the woman I loved, sculpted day by day by this brutal miracle medicine, sat in silence beside me.

If experience teaches anything, it's that this process never gets easier. But the anxiety does evolve. It shifts. It settles into a different shape—one you can carry without dropping. Eventually.

Here Comes the Boom

Wheeling Wendi out of the infusion room after treatment number three, we were both spent. While Wendi appeared to sleep through most of her infusion, I had no idea how restful that "sleep" really was. Still, beneath the exhaustion, something unexpected remained: hope. Like a stubborn ember in the ashes of a quieted campfire, it refused to go out. That buried ember willed us forward, kept us upright. As we drove home that Monday evening, I had no reason to believe I'd be seeing Mayo through the front windshield sooner than planned.

Once home, Wendi went straight to bed, no interest in food—particularly not anything that generated a metallic taste, which meant most everything. I followed, carrying crackers and an electrolyte-infused Yeti, helping her settle in. She fell into what looked like sleep, and I took a few moments to grab a snack, send some updates, and make a quick call to my guardian angel. Television had long since lost its appeal after the gut punch, so I scrolled news headlines in silence. An hour passed. The sentry kicked in. Time for the first temperature check.

Nothing could've prepared me—physically, emotionally, spiritually—for what came next.

The unicorn of chemo side effects made her full debut, crashing violently into our fragile new normal. When I walked in, Wendi was physically present but mentally absent. Her eyes stared blankly at the ceiling. Her teeth chattered. She repeated, in a whisper to no one, "So cold." Her frail body trembled uncontrollably. Later, she would describe it as bugs crawling under her skin.

Sentry mode. Full activation.

I ran through the checklist. First, the weighted blanket—something my guardian angel had encouraged me to keep close. It helped, briefly. But rigors, as we'd learn, scoff at comfort. No number of blankets could smother the chills. And this was just the beginning. Soon, nausea arrived. I sprinted for the bucket. Note to self: Next time, leave it by the bed. Always.

Back at her side, panic was not an option. I retrieved the thermometer—101 degrees. Not great, but still below the dreaded 102 that might send us back to Mayo. Cold compress. She cursed me when I pulled back the blankets, but it had to be done. The battlefield was set, and I had to stay in the moment.

From her nightstand—blessedly stocked the week before—I pulled the prescriptions. Two Tylenol. Zofran for nausea. Then, reluctantly, Demerol. I've never been a fan of narcotics, but this one was prescribed to manage rigors. It was time.

She took them, then laid back, fists clenched, staring into space, whispering, "So cold. So cold." Those two words pierced through me. I was powerless to soothe her. Rigors is the very definition of a cruel riddle: freezing from the outside in, burning from the inside out. My focus stayed on that fever. Still 101. Small win.

The image of rigors in full bloom burns deep. Her sunken eyes never moved, as if bracing for impact. Her fists never unclenched. She seemed completely unaware of my efforts—compresses, fluids, meds. It was her versus something we couldn't see or understand.

Then I remembered the last bullet in the chamber. I called Mayo. The on-call nurse listened carefully—mostly interested in her temp and whether she was holding down fluids. When I described the meds I'd administered, she encouraged me to continue, reiterated the 102 mark, and told me to call back or head in if it held.

Battle instructions delivered. Chamber empty. It was just us now. Mano a mano.

Compresses. Temp checks. Fluids. I peeled back more blankets despite her protests. Her skin radiated heat. She remained rigid, shaking, eyes fixed to the ceiling. Her fever hit 102. I stood on the brink of surrender—ready to drive her to the ER.

But then she kicked off the last of her covers, clenched harder, drank deeply, and dug in. Her strength recharged mine. Somehow, we made it through the night. And while I played my part, the victory belonged to her—my petite cheerleader, powered by sheer grit and stubbornness.

The week that followed mirrored a battlefield aftermath. She rarely left her bed. I delivered food she wouldn't eat, sat silently nearby, and pushed fluids like it was my sole job. She didn't complain, but I know I earned a few silent curses. By Friday, she stood. By Saturday, she ate—just a bit. By Sunday, she asked to take a short walk. Each small victory demanded celebration.

Only two things now stood between us and the next infusion: another blood draw and the return of the Sunday scaries.

The Number Four

The number four held meaning in our family. We had four incredible kids. It was Wendi's favorite number—worn proudly on her high school jersey. My son-in-law wore it in college and pro basketball. My son wore it in high school. As I wheeled Wendi in for chemo treatment number four, I silently hoped the number might offer some luck.

No sir.

As the IV tower delivered another cocktail of drugs into her already weakened body, I shared with our infusion nurse the horror of the rigors that followed treatment three. She listened closely, asked questions, then spoke with Wendi's care team. They approved a saline flush after chemo—hoping to kick-start hydration and reduce the intensity of rigors. It was compassionate. It was smart.

It didn't work.

We left that day tired and cautious. She slept on the ride home—an omen I should've taken more seriously. By 6:30, she was in bed. By 9:30, rigors returned with full vengeance. Eyes locked to the ceiling. Fists clenched. Teeth chattering. "So cold. So cold."

I deployed everything immediately—Tylenol, Zofran, Demerol. No hesitation. At 10, I called the nurse. She was surprised how quickly symptoms had escalated—especially given the saline flush. She called back after consulting with our oncologist.

But instead of more ammo, I received pressure: Do everything to avoid the ER. With her white blood cell count so low, the hospital could be a petri dish. Even a mild virus could be catastrophic.

That was a hell of a burden. Stay home, alone, in a war zone with no new tools—or risk the ER. Just saltines and a Yeti bottle left in my hands. I sat beside her, trembling from helplessness.

And then I remembered the movie *We Were Soldiers*, Mel Gibson shouting, "Broken arrow," the call you make when you're outgunned and surrounded, when every aircraft in range is diverted to save you, no matter the risk.

I hovered near that moment. Her fever approached 103. I was ready to scream it—*broken arrow.*

But Wendi stirred. She needed the bathroom. I helped her stand, then realized I was carrying her. Her skin was chalk white, her body limp. The bathroom light revealed the full impact of the chemo drugs deployed to save her, while slowly killing her: fragility so complete, she no longer resembled herself.

Mere Minutes Do Matter

Laying her gently back in bed, I saw it. Her eyes—unfocused. Confused. She barely knew where she was. Her body had nothing left. My stoic sentry armor cracked. I had nothing more to give. I had failed. Failed her. Failed the oncologist. Failed to keep her out of danger. But I felt with every ounce of conviction that we needed more tools. Professional care. Mayo.

She whispered, barely audible, that she wanted to stay home. But I couldn't allow it. We argued—but only for seven minutes. And I remember that time exactly, because of what happened next.

At minute eight, I carried her to the car. It was a twenty-minute drive to Mayo. At minute thirteen of our drive, as I looked over to reassure her, she was gone. Turns out, those seven minutes of uncertainty mattered.

She didn't stop breathing. But her eyes rolled back. Her head slumped left, held up only by the seat belt. Her face went slack. No response. No signs of awareness. Her body appeared lifeless.

The stoic sentry gave way to raw panic.

"Wendi!" I screamed. Nothing. My right arm braced her from falling further. My left hand gripped the wheel as I floored the accelerator. No speed limits. No red lights. Just fear. Just urgency.

Outside the ER, I didn't need to yell. They saw it. A wheelchair arrived before I even opened the door. She stirred slightly as they lifted her. Dazed. Confused. But alive.

Inside, it moved fast. Port accessed. Fluids delivered. Blood pressure low. Fever high. She was admitted quickly, likely because of her low white cell count. They wanted her far from the ER crowd.

Three bags of saline. Tests I can't remember. I wasn't observing anymore; I was just trying to breathe.

They told me she'd stay the night. And that I couldn't. COVID restrictions. For the first time since the gut punch landed, I would not be at her side.

I held her hand. Smiled through clenched grief. Then left.

Mental Parlor Tricks

Walking out of the hospital doors felt so unnatural, like I was leaving something behind and completely unsure of where I was going. The darkness hit me, telling me it was nighttime, but I barely noticed, standing frozen in place. I turned to look back at the building that now held her outside my grasp. As I slowly made my way to the car, completely forgetting where I had parked it, one thought inside me, in a place deep and previously impenetrable, arose: I was alone. Not permanently, thank God. But alone for the first time since the initial gut punch landed, which seemed like a lifetime ago. Not knowing what else to do, I drove straight home. Not because I wanted to. Not because I thought I was going to be able to find some rest. But merely because I had no idea where else to go and zero interest in going anywhere. Looking back, sleeping in the car near the building was likely the right answer, but it never occurred to me. Home it was.

After walking in, the house felt so wrong without her inside it. Despite the pictures, the familiar hum of the appliances, and a waiting, extremely disappointed poocher, the empty house felt just that. Empty.

I wandered about in a daze, exhaustion pressing down through my shoulders. Without her to check on, I really didn't know what to do with myself. After the shock of the drive to Mayo, my fight-or-flight mentality remained and seemed insistent on sticking around. Even in this quiet house, with her resting at Mayo a mere twenty minutes away, surrounded by healthcare professionals, I couldn't relax. And I wouldn't let down. So I mindlessly paced. Room to room. As I paced,

I checked my phone constantly for updates that never came. The night stretched on, nearly unbearable.

This was the first night I had spent alone since the gut punch arrived. This was a surreal night, a sentry with no one to watch out for. A night that came after a drive to the ER during which I thought I had lost her. A night spent alone with my thoughts. I felt like I had failed at every checkpoint. Those thoughts plagued me as the night stretched on.

Not feeling at all comfortable in our bedroom, a place in which battle-like conditions played out the night before, I found some comfort on our living room couch. Little did I know that this would become a place I would retreat to often, as the bedroom was no longer viewed as a place I could look to for rest and peace. Somehow, as I laid there, the poocher's rhythmic breathing nearby, sleep did find me. Temporary. Shallow. But enough for the time being.

I checked my phone for updates. None came. Still unsure if, in fact, yesterday really happened, I made a short walk into our bedroom. Wendi was not there. The extremely bad dream was apparently very real.

Before long, daylight would break, visiting hours would resume, and I could return to the only place I currently now belonged—firmly entrenched by her side. After arriving at Mayo, fully prepared to resume my post as her sentry, the doctors confirmed what appeared to be obvious: Her condition was brought on through a negative reaction to chemo. Not sepsis. Not an infection. Not a heart condition. Just the cruel side effects from drugs designed to save her.

Arriving at this conclusion allowed us to start the slow checkout process and leave Mayo early that evening. Upon returning home, while the extra fluids she had received certainly provided her with an energy boost, she retired directly to the bedroom and stayed mostly confined to bed until Friday of that week.

While she rested, I spent the week caught in a mental countdown, which seemed to be serving as a survival mechanism. Four treatments down, twelve to go. My mind was using this mental countdown to break up the seemingly unbearable into something more palatable.

That countdown suddenly became a sort of lifeline, a way to manage the unmanageable. Similar to staring incessantly at the clock on the IV tower during infusions, mental countdowns help trick our minds into moving forward when the weight of the journey feels like it should crush us. But these mental parlor tricks come at a cost.

Repeating the countdown clock to manage the unbearable means constantly looking past the present, placing all your focus and energy toward the finish line. It became a constant bargain with time, telling yourself, "Let me just get through this and then life can resume again." Past the pain. But also past the small, sacred moments that are always quietly unfolding.

By relying so heavily on this mental parlor trick and looking forward in countdown mode, we are robbing ourselves of our present. And what happens when a countdown ends? Normally, it is a simple answer. Another one begins. And a completely different, distant finish line seems to appear.

Through looking ahead and relying on a countdown clock to manage adversity, present day, precious moments, are often bypassed. These are moments that, once lost, are lost forever. As difficult as it can be to recognize in the moment, even in the darkest, most challenging of times, there are moments to be seen, felt, lived, experienced, remembered, and cherished. The mental countdown helps compartmentalize the seemingly unmanageable, taking our focus off the adversity and moving it toward a finish line. But what it does not do is guarantee an outcome. And it has absolutely no influence as to what is waiting for you on the other side.

In this way, the countdown clock is both a lifeline and a gamble. You can absolutely count down every chemo treatment, focusing on the final infusion, but that does nothing to guarantee remission is waiting after the last treatment.

Still, I couldn't stop. Four down. Twelve to go. I needed to believe in a finish line, even if the road there was paved with moments I'd never remember.

A Rock Takes Shape

As we continued to navigate our new normal, the patterns and coping strategies we had unconsciously adopted began to harden—solidifying themselves into our evolved daily routine. The Sunday scaries continued in full force, but their target shifted. We were no longer afraid of chemo ports or unknown chemicals deployed within a mysterious infusion room. Experience had dulled that edge. Now, the fear and anxiety turned its lens toward what came after treatment—the side effects that crept in like thieves after sunset and the toll they exacted on us both.

But the scaries weren't done evolving. They dug deeper and found new, creative ways to ensure Sunday-night sleep remained just out of reach.

Wendi had stopped eating—everything tasted like metal. Her energy faded with each passing day. Muscles withered from weeks being confined to a bed. With every treatment, she physically disappeared a little more. And that gave the scaries new ammunition: What if her bloodwork didn't provide her with the green light for treatment? What if her body simply refused to take on more harm, if her body had absorbed all it could handle and could go no further?

The terrifying reality we carried was that our efforts—every infusion, every battle with rigors, every sleepless night—might be in vain if the cancer outlasted her ability to continue. With each Monday blood draw, we held our breath, terrified that the dreaded red light might come, halting everything.

The scaries preyed on this. This knowledge. This fear. Every week they whispered, "What if the treatments don't work? What if the cancer outruns the cure? What if these side effects and the battle-like conditions they generate are all for nothing?"

As weeks five, six, seven, and eight rolled in and by, bringing with them more battles, more appearances by the unicorn, and more ways to deplete our energy and strength, the fear grew worse, compounding with each additional treatment. Monday blood draws, leading to the wait at the coffee shop to find out whether her body would receive the green light for the next treatment, brought increasing levels of anxiety as we waited to hear our fate. The idea of interruption—of losing momentum—felt almost as brutal as the diagnosis itself. Because it wasn't just about enduring future chemotherapy anymore. It was about earning the outcome. The pain and sacrifice simply had to mean something.

I'd become more capable at managing the unicorn's expanding portfolio of side effects. But despite our oncologist's firm guidance to avoid hospital visits, given her decreasing white blood cell count, we reluctantly returned—again and again. During the first ten weeks of weekly chemo treatment, I drove Wendi to the ER three times. On two of those three visits, she was admitted to the hospital overnight.

On paper, a 30 percent ER rate might read like a failure. Proof that I had not done enough to shield her from unknown infections that could linger within an ER atmosphere. But in the height of our ongoing battle conditions, when the fever was raging, dehydration was front and center, and blood pressure levels were dangerously low, this untrained and unskilled sentry was doing everything he could to keep her safe. And, sometimes, in my unskilled judgment, that mandated a trip to the ER, to find skilled support and more ammo to throw at the unicorn.

In this sentry's humble opinion, given the conditions we endured, I feel as though a 30 percent hospital visit percentage was nothing short of a miracle.

Given the odds stacked against her—the intensity of side effects, the volatility of her immune system, the tightrope we walked between collapse and survival—making it to week nine at all felt like a triumph. Maybe, just maybe, we weren't failing. Maybe we were defying odds. I guess only our oncologist knew the truth.

Week number nine was no different. Another COVID test.

Another blood draw. Another breath held at our coffee shop. Another green light. And another infusion, dripping more chemicals into the veins. This time, though, we had some help.

Our second-oldest daughter, Cassandra, the one that created a makeshift barber shop on our back patio, returned to Scottsdale to spend time with us. She brought with her a few sets of clothes, along with her Mama Bear quality—always quick to protect, to step in, to shoulder burdens without being asked. When she arrived and saw her parents, battle-worn, she sensed immediately how threadbare we'd become. We didn't have to say a word. She knew.

Cassey offered to be part of that week's infusion process. Tag team, if you will. The sentry and Cassey would rotate shifts, sitting beside Wendi as she endured the chemo drips. While I was not sure how I felt about exposing our daughter to this process, my tank was nearing empty. My mind was as exhausted as my body. I was running on autopilot, and for the first time in weeks, I exhaled. I wasn't going to be alone.

And for most of that day, it felt normal. Routine. Even hopeful. Nothing had transpired that would lead us to believe week nine would be materially different than prior weeks.

But hope has a cruel way of stepping aside at the worst possible moment.

Shortly after the infusion ended, while Cassandra and I waited and prepared to take Wendi home, something shifted. Suddenly, Wendi was disoriented. Confused. Her blood pressure crashed. The IV tower lit up, making all kinds of sounds.

Nurses heard these sounds and rushed into her infusion cubicle like a military unit. Voices raised. Orders barked. Cassandra and I were frozen, asked to step back into the hallway.

We stood there, completely paralyzed. On the other side of the half wall, my wife, Cassandra's mother—so recently upright, stable, and preparing to come home—was the epicenter of organized chaos. This time, we weren't at home, fumbling through battle conditions, equipped with so few tools. This time, we were in the hospital, and even the pros looked alarmed.

Later, they would explain: Her body had suffered a cumulative hypersensitivity to Taxol, one of the two chemotherapy drugs. Her immune system apparently had had enough and turned violently against this drug. The result? A reaction that mimicked a type of septic shock—blood pressure plummeting, organs at risk, chaos taking the reins.

But in the moment, with Cassey and I standing nearby, hearing the orders being barked while we were shielded from view, all we knew was this: Her body was shutting down. And it wasn't good.

Mayo's team of pros moved fast. IV antibiotics. Saline. Vasopressors. Words we'd never used in daily life now defining our new normal.

From the hallway, the sentry stood in absolute anguish, attempting to calm and soothe his emotional daughter, while standing helplessly, unable to aid his wife in any meaningful way. I felt completely useless, merely praying that the team at Mayo could bring Wendi back to us.

Nine weeks of this—of survival. Of chasing down any ways to help address side effects. Of praying constantly that Wendi's spirit could outlast her body's desire to collapse. And now, standing in the hallway and hearing the commotion from her infusion cubicle, it felt like it had all funneled into this moment—this silent hallway, this half wall separating us from catastrophe.

But then—somehow—it happened. They brought her back.

Not unscathed. Not unchanged. But back.

Bodies began leaving the infusion cubicle, and soon after, some equipment began retreating from the scene. Eventually, the only remaining Mayo team member was our infusion nurse. When she felt comfortable, she called for Cassey and I to return, to make the walk from the hallway to the infusion cubicle serving as a makeshift triage. Suddenly, the cubicle returned to its former self, and Wendi had Cassey and I by her side, where we belonged.

As we all breathed and tried to make sense of what had just unfolded, I could sense that our infusion nurse had run through her own set of emotions. She did her best to explain what had transpired, and I felt her shock and fear. When the adrenaline levels began to return to normal, we attempted to bring the conversation back to small talk. Nothing brings emotions down like small talk, even if you remain distracted. And that's when our infusion nurse gave Wendi the nickname that would stick, the nickname I have recited through these pages: Wendi was deemed the unicorn of chemo side effects. The nurse explained that she simply had not seen someone suffer—and survive—so many different chemo side effects, a body shutting down week after week, only to get off the mat and take more the next week. And this? This one sealed it.

She was the unicorn.

Weekly Treatments No Mas

Getting her home after that ninth treatment—after watching her body literally crash and slowly rally once again—was equal parts relief and heartbreak. They kept the unicorn overnight for additional observation, likely recognizing that we all desperately needed a moment to breathe. Looking back, I believe this was the closest we came to losing her during this journey.

The reaction to Taxol had depleted whatever reserve she had remaining. She didn't leave the bed for days. She barely sipped fluids. Ate almost nothing. She seemed to age a decade. Watching her physically unravel was gutting in a way I didn't know how to process or articulate. Her hair—what little remained—was nearly gone. Eyebrows, eyelashes, the features that had once framed her face had faded. Her skin, ghostly pale, hung loosely over her slight frame. Her eyes—that had always sparkled with unyielding determination—were sunken, dimmed, their light flickering.

And yet, on the tenth Monday morning since beginning her treatment, she somehow rose. Not with strength, not with energy, but with sheer will. And, somehow, against all odds, another green light to the infusion room came our way.

This time, more than any prior time, I was stunned. And proud beyond measure. It was as if she was willing her blood to meet the necessary metrics. And looking at her, it was incomprehensible that she could achieve this, week after week.

I wheeled her in for her final weekly infusion with a sense of reverence. Ten consecutive weekly treatments. Ten straight weeks of war. No breaks. I wasn't sure if any of the nurses expected to see us again, so soon. But here we were—exhausted, frayed, but not broken.

This tenth straight infusion was different. There was no Taxol this time—only Paraplatin. The reaction from week nine had eliminated any further exposure to the Red Devil's toxic twin. The infusion moved quickly. There was no drama, no curtain call. Just saline, Benadryl, chemo, slow drips, and silence. It felt like a small, sacred victory.

We both knew the road ahead wasn't finished. More chemo treatments loomed—four more, now spaced every other week. But this moment? This was a milestone. The end of our weekly hell. The end, so we thought, of our most relentless stretch.

As we drove home that evening, following treatment, we didn't say much. We never needed to. But the gravity of what had just been accomplished lingered in the quiet space between us. It was in the way she leaned against the seat belt. In the way my grip on the steering wheel relaxed, just slightly. We were taking our moment that we felt we had earned.

We knew what was waiting for us that evening: the aftermath. Even without the Taxol, we were fully expecting the unicorn to provide her form of drama. Fever. Rigors. Nausea. But this time, we also had something else: a gift. A full two weeks until the next treatment. A break.

A vacation of sorts, in the language of our new normal.

For the first time in ten weeks, there would be no infusion on Monday. No blood draw. No drip. No silent countdown on the IV tower. Just space. Space to breathe. Space to recover, to truly exhale, to heal—however temporary it was.

And we needed it. God, we needed it. So desperately.

Following our battle conditions that night, Wendi stayed in bed for most of the week ahead. But something was different. There was a flicker of anticipation, a faint sense that we might get one or two normal days before diving right back in.

We also had something circled, in a bright highlighter, on the calendar, an event that could not have come at a more appropriate time. The day we had decided to celebrate Mother's Day was approaching, and with it, we would be blessed with all four kids for the first time since the gut punch. Our son-in-law was also coming and, you guessed it, that lovely little granddaughter, our precious Olivia. Amid our new normal, this was certainly an event that we had been holding onto with a very tight grip.

By Friday, she had made the big move from the bedroom to the living room, always a small but seemingly monumental victory. Her eyes brightened a touch when the walls changed. She never said it, but I could tell: The bedroom had become too associated with pain, too layered in trauma. The living room still offered windows to our previous normal. Maybe, just maybe, this is why I had retreated to the couch too, even long after the treatments were behind us.

By Sunday, I was holding onto hope that, without an infusion looming on Monday, the scaries may offer a reprieve, a break from the constant torture.

No such luck. Instead, they grabbed onto new material.

Vacations Come in Many Forms

Moving toward every-other-week treatments wasn't merely a pause in the action. This was a lifeline. The gift ahead was not a traditional one. But in the strange currency of our new normal, we were being handed something priceless: the gift of time.

The plan we forged in our heads was simple: rest, recover, rebuild.

Physically. Emotionally. Spiritually. Because after ten weeks of being knocked down and dragged through unimaginable side effects that seemed custom-made to break her, we desperately needed a breath. A break.

And for the first time in months, we started to imagine that maybe—just maybe—breathing was still possible.

The conversation that week, whether she was in the bedroom or living room, was centered around our day chosen to celebrate Mother's Day. The kids. And dear Olivia. I think we were purposely refocusing our minds away from treatments, chemo, and side effects, inserting something much more positive in its place. Something sacred. Something pure. Family.

By that Friday, when Wendi emerged into the living room, spirits rose, even if energy levels remained low. But seeing Wendi look out the windows, as opposed to staring at a ceiling, was always a reason to celebrate the moment.

For both of us, the living room offered the illusion of peace. Softer light. Fewer ghosts. No closets in which monsters could be lurking. Just the simple move from one room to another had started to feel like a declaration of survival.

While Monday did not come with an appointment in the infusion room, it still came with an appointment, a rather large one, an in-person meeting with our oncologist—the wizard of Oz himself. This would only be our third time seeing him face-to-face since the treatment plan was described. But his influence had never been far. His name came up during every infusion. His decisions were echoed in every middle-of-the night nurse call. He was the constant voice behind the curtain—always present but rarely visible.

And so, with new material to use, the Sunday scaries whispered a new script: What will he say? Has anything changed? Will the plan hold? Does he have any results to share?

Questions led to uncertainty. Uncertainty turned into restlessness. Restlessness invited anxiety. And before long, it was 3 a.m., and we were both wide-eyed in the dark, physically exhausted by the many tosses and turns that had occurred.

The Great Oz Moves Outside the Curtain

Walking into the oncologist's office, it was not lost on me just how much Wendi's appearance had changed in the twelve weeks from our initial meeting with him. Boy, did that feel like a lifetime ago. As he had done previously, our oncologist arrived on time, bringing his same calm, compassionate, and patient approach. He quietly started firing questions her way. "How are you feeling?" "How are you holding up?" "Are you eating and drinking enough?" These were questions that friends and family would often ask, making us feel at ease.

He then launched into the next phase of her treatment. As he had said to two very naive people some many weeks ago, we would now receive chemo treatments every other week, deploying two new chemo drugs into her system. He also shared some unexpected news that had moved far from our radar. Wendi had been approved for an experimental trial to test how an immunotherapy drug, Keytruda, might work for patients with triple-negative breast cancer. Insurance would not cover these costly, experimental treatments, but he had discussed this with the pharmaceutical company, assuring us they would cover the costs as part of this experimental trial. While this had been on our radar early in our search for a medical team, we were now deep into treatment, and our vastly different outlooks on chemotherapy led to some obvious questions, mostly centered on possible side effects. After all, the oncologist was sitting with the unicorn of side effects, and while we were happy to be considered for a trial, we were also apprehensive.

Our oncologist, aware of her status and unicorn reputation, seemed confident that this immunotherapy drug would not come with the potential of additional side effects. After a long conversation, it was decided to add Keytruda to the treatment plan at the appropriate time, as designated by the oncologist. Then, without warning, Wendi blindsided me.

As the conversation was winding down, she brought up something that we had only briefly discussed, something I had been quietly but adamantly opposed to. She asked our oncologist about the possibility of completing her final four biweekly treatments in Boise, Idaho, our former home for thirty years. She explained the comfort she would gain by being so close to friends and family, allowing us to also spend time at our summer home in McCall, Idaho. I found myself wondering just where her motivation rested. Neither person showing any sign of wanting my involvement or opinion, I listened carefully.

Regardless of motive—and to this day, I still cannot determine what drove this request—the oncologist's compassion came through, and he had no problem with meeting her desire to complete treatments in Boise. He asked us to coordinate through both the nurses and the hospital administration team, in both locations, to work on schedules. He would place his stamp of approval on this shift and work in the background to do whatever was necessary to make this happen. He did, however, openly discuss and acknowledge the risks—the airport, flight, crowded spaces—of potential sources for exposure. It was not only Wendi and her low white blood count that he was concerned with. Additionally, the sentry, as the primary caregiver, could not place himself at risk of contracting something and bringing it back to Wendi. Provided that proper precautions were taken, with a very careful eye toward maintaining distance from others whenever possible, our oncologist saw no reason she could not finish her treatments in Boise.

With that, and a few explicit precautionary words about the potency of a new chemo drug she would soon be exposed to, the wizard of Oz disappeared behind his curtain. We would rarely see him again until after Wendi's post-chemo surgery.

Change of Venue

The drive home from Mayo that Monday was quiet—too quiet, even for us. We were both deeply processing everything. The new chemo drugs. The trial approval. Wendi's curveball.

Much like her attempt for a dinner out with friends, weeks and weeks ago, was she doing this for me? Did she think I needed a change, some socialization, time in a place that felt like our true home? Or was this about her—seeing friends and family, resting peacefully near the lake, getting a glimpse of our world that had existed before the gut punch arrived.

Or was it something else—something darker? These were the thoughts that were normally reserved for Sunday night, but here they were, coming out in the light of day.

Was she afraid it could be her last summer? Her last chance to be in McCall, to sit by the lake, to see the people she loved in the place where she felt most herself? Try as I might to suppress these dark thoughts, this possibility no doubt existed in both of our minds.

I was also processing the warnings about social distancing and remaining healthy, both of us, no matter what. If I got sick, even something minor, it could compromise everything.

She didn't bring up the plan to shift to Boise. Didn't push. She gave me space to process, which told me she knew it had landed hard.

And truthfully, this unilateral disruption to our treatment schedule could have shattered our unspoken agreement. We hadn't had a single fight since the diagnosis. The little things we used to bicker over had evaporated. Cancer had stripped all that away. But this? This could have risked breaking that streak.

I stayed quiet. She stayed patient. And, together, we let the silence do the work.

A quick lesson in geography would be appropriate here. Mayo, where treatments had been conducted, was twenty minutes from our home in Scottsdale. Boise, where treatments would now be conducted, was two hours from our summer home in McCall, Idaho. The two-hour drive from Boise to McCall was mostly journeyed on a divided, two-lane highway, with very little population along the path, and with very spotty cell service.

Over the next few days, I thought hard, attempting to do my

best to process every angle. And I kept landing in the same place: She had earned this. Every ounce of rest, every moment of comfort, every familiar face. She had endured the unimaginable—and she was still standing. If she wanted Boise, it would be Boise. If she needed McCall, it would be McCall.

But there was one piece of the puzzle ahead that I couldn't let go of. I desperately wanted, likely needed, her first biweekly treatment—the first round with the new chemo drugs—to happen at Mayo.

Not because I didn't believe in Boise. Not because I didn't trust the team there. But because Mayo knew her. Mayo had lived through the unicorn's side effects, logged every symptom, anticipated every twist. After so many years living there, Boise knew her name. But over the past months in treatment, Mayo knew her body.

I spent days working up how to approach this conversation with Wendi. I so did not want to disappoint her, nor upset her in any way. I stressed and agonized over this. I rehearsed lines in my head. Played out possible reactions. But when I finally brought it up—gently—she didn't hesitate. She agreed, instantly. No fight. No defensiveness. Just love. And with that, we would do her first biweekly treatment at Mayo. She would be exposed to these two new chemo drugs in a place, in an environment, that had become such a big part of our new normal.

And with that, we were fully back in sync.

While she rested that week, I moved into logistics mode. Hospitals, schedules, insurance, travel. I made phone calls. Sent records. Coordinated appointments across three locations: Mayo, Boise, and McCall. I even went as far as to schedule saline flushes to be administered at the small hospital in McCall, knowing elevation and dehydration could wreak havoc on the unicorn.

Every box I could check, I checked. Every contingency I could plan for, I planned. I also made a call I never imagined I would make.

I asked an individual who was blessed with the means to own a private plane for a rather large favor. I absolutely hated this ask. In our previous normal, such an ask would have never been considered. This felt like a favor simply too big to ever request. But flying commercial and navigating through airports seemed like an incredibly difficult burden to undertake. I was so reluctant to expose Wendi and myself to the chaos of airports, particularly in the post-COVID world. So many risks. So many people. So many unknowns. Not now. Not in her current state.

I was reluctant. I rehearsed the conversation. Over time, I built up courage. I had no idea how this request would be received. And, just like the conversation with Wendi, my reluctant request was met with an emphatic yes. No hesitation. No questions. True compassion still exists.

One more hurdle was cleared.

Still, even as everything fell into place, I held on to one final bit of anxiety. New drugs meant new unknowns. Unknowns meant anxiety. Anxiety meant no sleep.

Without Further Ado, Please Welcome the Red Devil

Our first biweekly infusion day started like the ten that had come before. COVID screening. Blood draw. Waiting for the green light to permit entrance into the infusion room. Despite the extra week of rest, we still felt the now-familiar flicker of unease as we waited.

She was cleared. The new chemo drugs were a go.

We met briefly with our oncology nurse for a quick review of the new plan. Two new chemo drugs, administered one after the other. No Taxol this time. Also, no turning back.

We were led to the infusion room and settled into our cubicle for the day. Saline flush. Benadryl. All routine by now. The first of the two new chemo drugs arrived, and everything seemed familiar. No immediate reactions. No surprises. No sirens.

All that changed when the second bag arrived. This one looked . . . different. Remarkably, noticeably, visibly different.

Violent. Bright red. Like the chemical in the bag had no business being inside a human body. The nurse hung the bag on the IV tower, and it suddenly appeared in our lives, like a warning. Looking up at the bag above, only one thought came to mind: Buckle your seat belts.

I glanced at Wendi. She looked at me. No words were exchanged—but we both thought the same thing: What the hell is that?

Our nurse, suited up in hazmat-style gear, approached with casual precision. "This one's doxorubicin," she said. "You may have heard of it by another name—the Red Devil."

Yep. We had.

The name didn't sound clinical like Paraplatin or Paclitaxel. It sounded, instead, like a warning. Like folklore. Like something whispered behind closed doors. It sounded personal. Violent. Vicious. Like it had earned its reputation one patient at a time.

The timer was turned on and the drip was set to begin. And I stared, unblinking, watching the bag, frozen, almost hypnotized. That liquid red, winding its way in the IV tube, dripped slowly toward her veins. It felt wrong. It didn't belong in her body. It looked corrosive, like it could burn through steel.

I couldn't look away. And worse—I couldn't trust it.

I sat silent and still. Every instinct screamed for me to act, rip out the IV tube, stop this red liquid from reaching her veins, heart, brain, bones. But I didn't. I couldn't. I was the sentry. Only act when called upon. Don't stop the war. Silently stand post while it raged around me.

The contents of that red bag eventually entered Wendi's system, traveling quietly but relentlessly, seeping into every corner of her body until no cell remained untouched. Then, graciously, came the posttreatment saline flush. That clear liquid—pure and familiar—felt like a rescue mission. A giant neutralizer. As if it might rinse away whatever evil had just been delivered. Maybe. Hopefully. A cleanse and a healing.

The Devil's Aftermath

We left the infusion center composed but deeply unsettled. We were veterans who thought we knew what to expect. But this time, it was different. There was a new energy between us. Apprehension. Tension.

Something in the air had changed. The Red Devil was now inside her. However brutal prior side effects had been, this felt different. The unicorn never left treatment without bringing something unexpected home. It didn't take long to find out.

Within hours of returning home, the rigors returned, hard and fast. I'd seen Wendi shake before. I'd seen her teeth chatter and fists clench and eyes go vacant. But this was different. Her eyes and teeth had a reddish tint. It wasn't lighting or imagination. It was chemical. The Red Devil had come home with us—not just metaphorically. Visibly. Like it had marked her.

That was when it really hit me: This damn drug was in everything. It was in her bloodstream, her breath, her sweat, and now staining our sheets. Earlier in treatment, the nurses had quietly warned me: Be cautious. Don't share a bed. These drugs aren't just tough on patients. They can be toxic to caregivers too. But it felt hypothetical. Not anymore.

And yet, in the thick of battle, I couldn't think about self-protection. I needed to stay in the fight, take temperatures, cycle through meds, and be near her to whisper reassurances while she clenched her jaw and begged through chattering teeth for warmth she couldn't feel. I threw everything available to me within my growing arsenal at her rigors: Tylenol, Zofran, Demerol, layers of blankets, and cold compresses. There was no sleeping that night. Not for her. Not for me. These were full battle conditions, as we made every effort to keep her out of the hospital. This wasn't about recovery. That would come, perhaps, one day. This was just about survival.

By morning, we hadn't gone to the hospital. This should have felt like a win. But it didn't. Her body was wrecked. Destroyed in new ways. This round, the wounds had cut deeper.

Armed with limited tools, Wendi's deep reservoir of resiliency was perpetually tested.

The unicorn displayed symptoms that lingered longer than anything we'd seen before. But we braced. Adjusted. Adapted. Her sentry stayed on high alert, managing each hour as it came. Fluids and food were a must, but to her, everything tasted like aluminum. Even water had a metallic tang. Every meal became a negotiation, and the sentry rarely won.

Then I remembered the box. My guardian angel had warned me in his own quiet way. Knowing the Red Devil was about to join the party, he sent me a box, telling me to "only open if necessary." The phrase hinted at what contents may be inside. I hadn't touched it. Until now.

After breaking the seal, I found celery juice—fully expected, familiar, already part of our playbook. Keep her hydrated. But tucked alongside it were items I didn't understand. Swabs. Numbing gels. Tools and items you'd expect in a dentist's office, not in a cancer battle kit.

At first, I assumed these were for the red tint in her mouth, a reaction to the drug's hue, maybe. I wish that had been the case. Instead, we were about to meet yet another cruel gift from the Red Devil: mouth sores. Not just little ulcers or irritations. These were large, aggressive, blistering wounds. Painful to the point of tears. They made speaking difficult and swallowing unbearable. And chewing? Out of the question. The unicorn took it straight on.

The care box helped. The swabs, the gels, and the cooling rinses all did their part in offering some sliver of relief. But these sores did not burn out in a day or two. They lingered. They deepened. And while her taste buds had already made eating a chore, now the act itself became a source of suffering. Food appeared to be off the table for a while, not out of nausea or disinterest, but because it simply hurt too much to eat. That week stretched on. No hospital visit, but still hell. And over that week, I watched her fade.

Not all at once. Slowly. In fragments. Her movements were more cautious. Her sleep—when it came—was light and fractured. Every shift in bed required effort. Every sigh, a calculation. Every wince, more noticeable.

With the power of the Red Devil deposited within her veins, her body was in a constant tug-of-war with the various side effects. The sheets were no longer merely fabric. They were evidence. The stains became records of what she was enduring. Proof of what had passed through her.

And I saw something else that week.

In her eyes, there was a new glaze. Not just exhaustion. Not just pain. Something much deeper. She blinked slower. Stared longer at nothing. She tried to hide it—but I knew. I knew she was fighting pain in her mouth every time she closed it. I knew she was facing a bully with few limits, on energy levels that did not make this a fair fight.

She tried to smile for me. Tried to walk. Tried to act like all was well. But the smile didn't reach her eyes.

And then there was me. Something started to bubble up in me that week. Something I didn't want to name. A feeling I was not expecting, a feeling I had not trained for.

Fear.

Damn it. With all my energy, focus, and attention fixed on the battle, this was not a feeling I'd known before. Not this kind of fear. It wasn't fear that she wouldn't survive the week, though that thought did cross my mind. No, it was the fear that I was watching something unravel that I couldn't control or repair, even with my newfound skills acquired during this new normal. The Red Devil was asking me to stay fully present, fully engaged—and still accept that I couldn't save her from this part of our journey. The intense fear that I felt, for the first time, came directly from feeling completely powerless.

Helpless and terrifying as it was, I buried it, like all the rest. That's what a sentry does. Emotions weren't tools. They were distractions.

So I watched. I stayed close, almost hovering. I took her temp. I adjusted pillows and encouraged fluids. Monitored every flicker of her discomfort. I dimmed lights. Turned down voices. I did everything I could to make sure she didn't feel like she was missing out on life.

Even as I began to suspect . . . she already had.

Homeward Bound

After the Red Devil had scorched its way deep into our lives and the worst of that round's aftermath began to fade, a new chapter quietly emerged. While not a clean break, this would result in a change in light, in air, in the shape of our day. Boise was about to alter our existing patterns. We were about to go home. Where loved ones awaited, a community. Home.

Wendi's insistence on continuing chemo treatments in Boise felt both necessary and symbolic. In her opinion, the only one that truly mattered, she needed a place to deeply rest, one where I could find some help. She wanted fresh eyes, new hands, and people who didn't see her as a medical chart, but as Wendi, mother of four. While I remained apprehensive, she was embracing this. Wanting this. Needing this. She saw this change in scenery bringing freshness, a new infusion room, a different rhythm, and a new kind of quiet. For her, I had to play all in.

We both understood that her cancer would not retreat merely because we changed zip codes. That being said, I definitely noticed a shift. Wendi, still hollowed out by her aggressive treatments, began to gather herself differently. Carefully. She moved like someone trying to recall what her former self looked like, before chemo had taken so much of her vitality. Her body was still fragile, still raw from the inside out, but something much deeper was stirring. Like perhaps, just perhaps, the unicorn had found a sliver of safe ground to stand on again.

It took me time to understand that her decision was influenced by the people in Boise and the majestic scenery in McCall. After reaching McCall, this second part became easy to understand. The nearby mountains now framed our mornings. The smell of pine brought us possibility and hope. Even the smaller hospitals felt different. Gentler. While it could have been the staff, it was more likely just being back in a place that had always felt like our refuge.

Lasting Memories on a Postcard

The dramatic change in scenery and the fresh mountain air, coupled with the eight days until our first chemo treatment in Boise, emboldened Wendi to make yet another unilateral decision. While my need to protect her made me apprehensive again, I instinctively knew her decision could not be changed. Rather than hesitate or discuss, I jumped in without even a blink. If she needed this, perhaps I did as well. We had a tradition of playing in a charity golf tournament in McCall for twenty-five years, which helped to support the local McCall community. Even in her current physical condition, she so passionately believed that our participation in this annual event would remind us, if even for a day, what normal used to look like.

Then came the day. Skies so blue, we felt we were living within a postcard. Early summer light. That soft McCall breeze that always seems to know just when to show up. For longtime McCall residents, this day had long been viewed as the kickoff for summer, and the weather on this day did its part.

We joined incredibly close, supportive friends for our annual round of golf to support the McCall community. These were wonderful souls who knew her deeply, who had passed along prayers and waited for any word over the long, punishing weeks and months of treatment. This day had more meaning, as so many of the folks who would see her had not seen her since the gut punch. Crazy how something like cancer doesn't really seem real until you see, for yourself.

With our dear friends with whom we play annually in this event, we designed the day to be a gentle outing. Wendi would ride along in the cart, nothing more. Along with my close amigo, who played college basketball and possesses a larger-than-life presence within the community, we would stand guard over Wendi, making sure proper distance was maintained and, God forbid, no one moved in for a hug. She would watch the game and feel the sun, breathe in some mountain air, and embrace what our normal used to look and feel like.

Eighteen holes later, which meant five-plus hours in a charity tournament, Wendi had done something that none of us had expected: She stayed. For someone who had rarely left the bedroom, much less the house, for nearly five months, staying outside with loved ones on that now memorable day was an absolutely remarkable feat. It was even more impressive, considering it was still amid treatment and with the Red Devil lurking around the corner. Truly astonishing. No one paid attention to the game or kept score. All eyes were on her. She rode along, laughed, chirped in with commentary, and joined in on stories in between shots. And her smile . . . God, her smile. It wasn't the practiced one she had worn to get through appointments. It wasn't the tired one she quickly flashed to nurses when she thanked them for poking her with needles. This smile was different. This one was authentic. This was Wendi's real smile.

And her eyes seemed to smile just as brightly. For the first time in what felt like forever, those amazing eyes shone and matched the smile on her face. That moment on the golf course, under that sky, with those people, became our emotional summit. Birth of kids. Nope. Graduations and marriages. Nope. Selling a business. Nope. That moment. That smile. That feeling of pure triumph during an enduring battle against something you couldn't see. Our battle was far from over, and we both knew that. But that day gave us something that had been taken away from us: joy. Unfiltered. Unmasked. Undeniable. We both knew, without saying it, that we would carry that day with us. Like a flask of warmth tucked away for the remaining cold days ahead. A battery we'd draw strength from. A reason and an enduring memory to help stay in the fight.

The Red Devil Does Travel

Even with all our efforts to pivot—changing landscapes, adjusting plans, building hope around a new medical team—distance and new zip codes didn't spare us from the infamous Red Devil. That brutal drug found us again, right there in Boise, waiting patiently for the next round. Wheeling Wendi into the infusion room was similar, yet different. The room was much smaller, darker, more compact. There were no private cubicles, just infusion chairs set out in a shared space. And yet, somehow, there was a similar energy. The staff made it that way. While they were without the bells and whistles of Mayo, warmth radiated from the staff, bringing energy to the dark room. You could tell they cared, and that is all that mattered.

During infusion number fourteen, Wendi rested, eyes half closed, allowing the IV to drip its fluid into her veins. I sat in a small chair beside her, back in my usual role: watchful, alert, quietly taking inventory. The drips moved along, and time slowed in that strange way it always does in infusion rooms. Then, the infusion nurse leaned toward me, soft-spoken but curious. She began asking questions about Mayo, that mysterious place where research was conducted and brilliant minds coexisted, wrapped in clinical legend. She was hungry for insight—not out of comparison but curiosity, wanting to understand what Wendi had already endured.

She peppered me with follow-up questions, especially regarding the aggressive and compact treatment schedule. How was she holding up? What side effects had she experienced? What had we seen? I gave her some of it, enough to be honest and helpful. But not the full story. No chance for the full story. By now, I had become an expert at swallowing memories and visuals before they made it to the surface. The chattering teeth. The red stains. The mouth sores. The fever spikes. The stressful sprints to the ER. Most of this was tucked away, packed deeply to avoid the reality, allowing me to stay vigilant and alert. Had I shared these reels with our compassionate nurse, I am not sure she would have believed me. I lived them and still question them even today.

The nurse listened intently, her brow creasing in moments of concern. But she never looked away. She told me, earnestly, that she would do everything in her power to help minimize side effects. She'd push hydration, adjust timing of drips, offer meds, keep a close watch. I believed her intentions were nothing but pure. Her care, real. But there was one truth she didn't yet know: Boise hadn't yet met the unicorn in full bloom. And there seemed to be no protocol for that.

Skipping the Line Again

We were soon tested again. Damn that Red Devil. No amount of blue skies or mountain air could hold back the storm that followed round fourteen. If this were a boxing match, they certainly would have thrown in the towel. The unicorn was absolutely introduced to Boise. By force. By fever. By collapsing into my arms in an elevator and shocking a poor soul waiting innocently, his normal unexpectedly colliding with ours.

When our elevator ride reached the lobby, chaos spilled out as the doors opened. A stranger, wide-eyed and frozen, held the doors open as I gathered Wendi into my arms. He followed us out, helping to steady her legs as I half-carried, half-pulled her to the car. We left him standing on the sidewalk, still stunned, as we sped away.

Leaving him behind didn't mean our panic subsided. On the contrary, it rode with us—heavy, breathless, and unrelenting—all the way to the hospital. Damn that Red Devil. We had escaped the elevator but not the descent.

At that moment, the ER was packed. Overflowing. The receiving nurse, clearly overwhelmed, heard our information and asked us to wait. In a crowded room filled with coughs, infections, and viruses. A room that would be a mild inconvenience to most, but to someone with a severely compromised immune system and a body drowning in side effects, it was a minefield.

The unicorn could not wait. And, therefore, neither could her sentry.

Something had clearly changed in me. I wasn't the hesitant, deferential man I had been, still learning what it meant to take point. No, by now, I knew exactly what she needed and, more importantly, how to get it. No reason to wait in a crowded room. No need for tests or triage. The unicorn needed fluids and Benadryl, and she came complete with a port access.

I wheeled her straight out of the ER and across the hospital, bypassing the chaos, moving not with arrogance but with hard-won clarity. She didn't need a bed or a night in the hospital. She needed a chair. And an IV tower. Hydration was crucial. And we needed that infusion nurse—the one who, just the day before, had looked me in the eye and promised she'd do everything she could to ease Wendi's suffering. I had no appointment. No referral. Just a compromised wife and a fierce belief in what she needed.

There was some initial confusion when we arrived at the infusion room. Some sideways glances. A good amount of hesitation. Ignoring this, I calmly but firmly explained what had happened, what I believed would help, and told them to call Mayo's oncology department if they needed reassurance. Within minutes, we were ushered in and welcomed by that same nurse from the day before, displaying the kind of rare grace that cannot be taught. She got to work immediately. Fluids flowed. Relief followed. Wendi leaned back in her chair, her confusion subsiding, and the storm began to lift, if only momentarily.

And now the unicorn was properly introduced to Boise. Not in theory. Not through charts or plans or descriptions. But face-to-face. And now this graceful, compassionate nurse understood: This fight wasn't clinical. It wasn't theoretical. It was deeply human. Messy. Urgent. Real. Our infusion nurse may have learned something that day. I know I did. I learned that I was not there to follow the rules. I was there to help my wife survive. Even if that meant cutting the line on occasion.

Sequels Rarely Deliver Like the Original

Once Wendi could tolerate the winding two-hour drive back up into the mountains, we returned to McCall. It wasn't so much a retreat as it was a strategic withdrawal. Her body needed rest. Real rest. And space to recover from its second encounter with the Red Devil.

She was limp. Hallowed. A warrior with limited rations who was clearly battle-fatigued and worn down to the bone. After spending a few days in McCall, days in which she never left her bedroom, our summer retreat felt different. McCall, our healing place and our sanctuary, felt off. Muted. The trees were still emitting their piney scent, and the lake still shimmered with each change in the light, but the energy had shifted. Summer had arrived, but it might as well have been mid-July in Scottsdale. Hot. Heavy. Still.

She spent most of that week following treatment in bed, staring up at the ceiling. I don't think she noticed the fan slowly spinning above, moving air throughout the room. I think she was staring through it. Past it. Looking toward something only she could see.

Her finish line. In whatever form she imagined it to look like.

She didn't say it. She never discussed this. She didn't need to. After everything, I could feel it. Her silent stare was not signaling surrender; it signaled strategy. She was conserving energy, mentally bracing herself for the final push. She was willing her blood counts to rise. Willing her body to hold just enough to get her through the second-to-last treatment. Her next rendezvous with the Red Devil.

And I, her sentry, did what I always did in these in-between spaces: I paced. I watched. I overanalyzed. I calculated when and how much she drank. I tracked her skin tone, the glassiness in her eyes, the quiet of her voice. I refreshed prescriptions, ensuring our ammunition was properly stocked. I fielded some texts, updating people I did not want to worry, hoping word would spread. I took her to the small, intimate McCall hospital for fluids. Again. And again. And again.

But the miracle of the day on the golf course, that moment when the sky had opened and her spirit had peeked through? It was slipping further into memory with each drip from the IV tower. Like a postcard from a trip we once took. A place I wasn't sure we'd get back to.

And though I had worked hard to build this bridge to Boise and had placed so much hope in a new team, a new place, and a fresh start, I began to feel a gravitational pull back south. Back to the rhythm we had grown so accustomed to. Back to the Mayo team that had seen Wendi at her worst and built the battle plan that had gotten us this far. Back to where this journey, this quest, had started. While rest was vital and the mountains were healing, our moment on the golf course had passed, and I strongly felt the safest way to finish this journey was to return to the course we started on.

Speed Bumps Come in All Sizes

I started quietly preparing for a return to Mayo, building a plan in my mind, packing bags that hadn't been unpacked for long, and sorting out the journey. I also knew Wendi was not ready for this. Not even close to ready.

She was still holding tightly to that single, spectacular day on the golf course, clinging to it with vice grips. She wasn't ready to let that go. Not yet.

So when I casually floated the idea of heading back to Scottsdale, it didn't take more than her eyes for me to understand her thoughts. We were staying. For now. And this was her fight.

The time until her next treatment passed slowly. She was not showing signs of regaining her physical strength, spending much of the time in bed. But you could see her, as time passed, begin to psyche herself up, building her resiliency to mentally will her way into that infusion room. Eventually, like time always does, it passed, and we made the two-hour ride back to Boise. Back toward the dark, intimate infusion room, where privacy was more suggestion than reality.

For fourteen consecutive treatments, we had managed to thread the needle. No matter how gaunt she looked, how empty her energy tank appeared, the green light always came.

But not this time. Irrespective of the change in zip code, this time, she could not will her way past the blood draw results. This time, a red light came her way. Prior to treatment number fifteen, so achingly close to the end, we found a rather large speed bump, and there would be no treatment on this day. The Red Devil would have to wait. Her blood counts were simply too low.

We were quickly on the phone with Mayo. The wizard of Oz was pulling levers with speed and precision. But this lever, once we heard the plan, tugged at us emotionally in a way that even chemo hadn't. This was a lever not about poison but about life. To keep her moving forward, Wendi would need something she'd never needed before: a blood transfusion.

It was jarring and unexpected.

It's hard to explain what these words do to you when you first hear them, not as a headline or an abstract concept but as a necessity. It felt invasive. A quiet reminder that this wasn't just a battle against cancer anymore. This was a fight to keep her body fueled, functioning, and upright. We simply had to make it to the next round, whatever it took.

No tubes that day carried chemo. Instead, an unknown stranger's blood coursed into Wendi's veins, another anonymous gift, another form of hope. And strangely, this was a reset. While this was not the day we had planned, it was the day her body needed. Because when you are that close to the finish line, you don't look for shortcuts. You look for strength.

Back to the Land of the Cactus

Her incredibly deep reservoir of resilience carried the day, again. Just a few days after her blood transfusion, her numbers began to rebound. Not dramatically. But enough. Just enough to earn the green light for chemo treatment fifteen. This would be our last treatment in Boise.

We returned to the dark infusion room, sat with our extremely compassionate infusion nurse, and welcomed back the Red Devil. But that was not the headline of the day. The real headline was "Wendi Made a Decision." She suddenly saw things my way. Not because I pushed but because the blood transfusion immensely shook her. She was all in and ready for a return to Mayo.

Her focus was to finish what we started and complete the journey in the very place where our normal had first unraveled. To go back with deliberate intent, because some things deserve to end in the place where they began.

With that decision made, we began our journey home. Or rather, a journey to the place we had come to understand as our "home base" in our long battle against triple-negative breast cancer. Through the compassion and generosity of another good friend, we returned to Scottsdale by private plane—a journey that would not have been possible otherwise. After landing at a small airport in Scottsdale, I looked at her and deeply appreciated her desire to return to Boise. If only for a short period. I think that day on the golf course gave her the grit to handle more interaction with the Red Devil, eventually landing us back where her journey could be completed.

Helping her down from that plane was a moment I will never forget.

It felt sacred. Quiet. Unseen by the busy world around us. She moved slowly down the short stairs. But she moved, and that was enough.

We were met at the airport by a dear friend, the same one who had once carried her out of a restaurant after her body collapsed in protest. That episode felt like a lifetime ago, but the love and loyalty of our dear friend remained unchanged, even within this new normal. And just like that, twenty minutes later, we were fully back in Arizona. Back in the place where the unicorn had first revealed herself. Where the gut punch had landed. Where her tears first fell in the infusion room. Where we learned how to surrender and fight in the same breath.

And we both felt comfort in knowing that we were just twenty minutes away from Mayo. The place where it all began. Where chemo number sixteen was waiting—sixteen of sixteen. And a place where we would have our final interaction with the Red Devil.

Time to Fill the Balloons

It felt like a weight was being lifted. But simultaneously, you could feel another quieter, heavier weight settling in. We were near the end of her plan. There were no more drugs left to try. No more Red Devils hiding in the bushes. The kitchen sink had been thrown and landed.

And as she quietly rested through that final infusion, surrounded by familiar faces and with bright sunshine pouring through the large windows, I felt something loosening in my chest. The coil that had been wound tighter and tighter with every treatment began, for the first time, to ease. Ever so slightly.

When the IV pump clicked off for the final time, balloons appeared. Yes, balloons. And smiles broke out among the medical team carrying in these balloons. A few "You did it" cheers came from the nurses who had so professionally cared for her along the way. But while Wendi emotionally accepted this cheer and fellowship, something was not lost on me. This wasn't just a victory lap. This was it. Not the last treatment in some linear schedule. The last treatment available to her. We had reached the edge of the medical road map.

We left Mayo that day quieter than we had walked in. Not in defeat but in deep, exhausted reverence. Because somehow—*somehow*—she made it. She endured sixteen treatments, countless side effects, rigors that shook her bones, sprints to the ER, and allergic reactions that nearly claimed her life. She made it through every punch that cancer sent her way, even when her body had nothing left to give. The balloons we carried to the car proved it. Her infusion treatments were over.

Now, the only thing left to do was wait. To rest. To heal and to hope. And to pray. A lot. Because the treatment chapter was closed. The fight had been fought. The poison had been delivered. But the results?

The results were waiting in the distance, hidden just out of reach, making us hold our breath while the healing began.

The Silence After the Storm

Time, which had dragged its feet throughout the chemo treatment schedule, now felt like it was stuck in molasses. We weren't sprinting anymore. No rushing to appointments. No tracking nausea cycles or chasing fevers with saline bags and Benadryl. Just silence. And an open calendar.

No treatments. No blood draws. No schedules. And in that silence, the noise in my head grew louder. The unicorn had emptied every chamber during her final appearance. She had gone out swinging, throwing every last side effect like one final tantrum. And somehow, we had withstood it. That endurance gave us a small, quiet amount of confidence. Not the kind you talk about or even admit to yourself, but the kind you cling to at 3 a.m. when fear claws into your spine.

Now, we shifted into the hardest phase yet: the waiting. Surgery was the next milestone on the calendar. This was a single day that would mean everything. The double mastectomy. The cosmetic reconstruction. And between these two separate surgeries, the removal and the rebuilding, we would have *the* moment. The one moment that every treatment, every setback, every sleepless night was building toward.

Because in that space between surgeries, results would be uncovered. Lymph nodes would be harvested. Margin tissue would be removed and examined, the battlefield surveyed.

Had the Red Devil done its job? Had the tumors surrendered? Had the cancer spread? All we could do was wait. And wonder.

Wendi rested in those long weeks, her body slowly regaining its strength. But rest doesn't always mean peace, especially not when a date is circled on the calendar that could so define our future. Every night during that time felt like a Sunday. And it wasn't just the fear of Monday. It was the fear of everything.

This was the hush before the reveal. The inhale before the verdict. The calm before the storm. And in that stillness, we held on to each other tightly. Carefully. Waiting for the verdict.

The Envelope, Please

The day finally found us. The long wait was over. It was surgery day. *Results* day.

A close friend with some medical experience generously offered to fly down from Boise to support Wendi with post-surgery care. We had been told there would be drains to manage, and even a sentry has limitations. Without hesitation, our friend boarded a flight, eager to lend a hand and be with us when the results dropped.

That morning, we woke with a strange mix of apprehension and anticipation. Like it or not, we were about to find out. Everything. We drove to Mayo early, heading straight to pre-op. We had only met our oncology surgeon once before, but she greeted us with the same calm confidence. Though clearly busy, she took the time to walk us through every step of the surgery. She then carefully took my phone number, promising to call when she had news. We both knew what that meant.

After answering a few questions, she told me to hug my wife before she was wheeled into the OR. And with that, still holding on to my sentry role, I looked at Wendi, deeply shoved my emotions into the same overflowing hole I'd been using for months, and told her everything was going to be okay. As she was wheeled away, I stayed motionless, realizing our wait was officially almost over.

I returned home, gathered our friend, and invited two more of Wendi's closest friends to breakfast. The four of us sat at a table, ordering plenty and eating almost nothing. Our minds were elsewhere—waiting on the call that could define everything.

Tick. Tick. Tick.

Boom.

Out of nowhere, the phone rang. I answered without thinking, walking away from the table, needing both quiet and distance. For a moment, the call felt awkward, like watching an award show where everyone knows the envelope holds the answer, but small talk still permeates. She handled the surgery well. The reconstruction was already underway. The nipple-sparing portion looked good and would likely result in minimal scarring. Yada. Yada. Yada. That is what I remember, but there was likely more.

Then came the results, delivered straight toward a head that was already spinning.

The lymph nodes showed no signs of cancer. No signs of spreading.

Breathe. Wait.

She moved on to the margins—clean. No sign of cancerous cells outside the tumor areas.

Breathe. Still more.

As for the tumors, they hadn't just shrunk. They had evaporated. Vanished. She didn't have to remove them—they were already gone. Completely gone.

Then she spoke in my language: "This was an absolute home run." The chemo hadn't just worked—it had eliminated the cancerous cells. No signs of spreading. No remaining cancer cells. A rare result. And you could hear genuine excitement in her voice.

Holy shit.

I thanked her more times than I could count, forgot to ask when Wendi would be out of surgery (a nurse would later call), and hung up.

I wanted to scream, climb a mountain, and go pure Rocky Balboa, yelling, "Yo, Wendi, we did it." But I chose a quieter, more manageable path. I walked quickly back to the table. Everyone's anxious eyes stared into mine. For a second, all emotions remained sealed up. I started, "That was the doctor . . ."

That's as far as I got.

Every emotion I'd crammed down during my time as a sentry blew out all at once. Tears. Deep, body-shaking sobs. The kind I couldn't speak through. I'm sure I scared them—they'd never seen me like that. After a few minutes, I summoned the strength to say, "We're good. Really good."

And that was enough. They didn't need to hear details about margins and lymph nodes. They needed to hear that their friend was good. After that, we made quite a scene at the restaurant. Smiles. Hugs. Tears. Laughter. We had no concern about how we looked; our spirits were lifted, and we took the moment to celebrate. Napkins were passed around like confetti, signaling a generous tip for the servers.

I stepped away, far away, to make some calls. Kids. Check. More tears, more celebration. Couldn't keep it together on those calls. The sentry had officially left the building. More calls. Loved ones and close friends. Check and check. While I had been blessed to feel pure joy, this feeling was unique. Exhaustion and emotions being crammed down internally for so long proved to be an interesting mix with elation. This was pure and rare. This was joy.

Back at the table, my heart was pounding nearly out of my chest. We sat and talked, literally reminiscing about the scene that just played out, everyone sharing their feelings. No one wanted to leave. Not wanting to be alone, I suggested we head to the mall together. They looked at me like I was nuts, as they knew me well enough to know the mall was not my scene. Time to ad-lib and roll out a plan. Each of them could pick out one thing for Wendi. Once she was not loopy from the meds and fully recovered from surgery, we would have her open the gifts, and she could select her favorite one to keep. By the way, they took full advantage of my spirits and added their own rule. No price limit. Done. The mall it was.

That afternoon was nothing but joy. Smiling. Crying. Being in the moment. Oh yes, and abusing my credit card.

Eventually, I had to say goodbye, leaving them with the gifts and memories we would always share. I had to go. I had someone to pick up at Mayo. Someone I couldn't wait to share some unbelievable news with.

Standing beside her bed at Mayo following surgery, tears streamed down my face. I am not sure Wendi fully grasped the magnitude of the amazing news just yet—her body fogged from the anesthesia following a day-long operation—but she could see it in my eyes. She didn't need words. She knew it was good.

As we stayed in recovery, both surgeons came by, each recapping their portion of the day, walking us through the next steps for recovery, and, most memorably, beaming with genuine happiness. Their work had led to something extraordinary, and they knew it. You could see it in the way they smiled, in the way they lingered just a little longer than they had to. They were proud. They were moved.

Then, finally, the last visit of the day: the wizard of Oz himself.

Our oncologist. He was no longer just a doctor. He was now family. And entrance into that circle didn't come easily.

He stayed with us longer than I would have ever expected. Likely longer than he had planned. He repeated the good news for Wendi, slowly and clearly, allowing it to land in her foggy post-op mind. And then he just sat with us. No rush. No clipboard. No questions. Together, we smiled. We cried. We said very little because, for the first time since the gut punch, there was nothing more to say.

He didn't need to say it out loud. You could just feel it: This mattered to him too.

Normalcy—Table for One

Elation rolled with us from Mayo, filling the house where battles were waged—even through the pain of recovery. The news had been miraculous. The surgery had gone better than expected. But despite the celebration and relief, the road ahead would still be long.

Both surgeons had worked their magic, but Wendi's body had a new challenge now: healing. Recovery was certainly not immediate, and it would not be easy. For months, she had to work through the tight grip of internal scarring. Every small stretch, every minor movement, was a reminder of what her body endured. The drains, the stiffness, and the limitations were all a quiet daily struggle, hidden beneath the noise of our gratitude.

Recovery didn't come with a fanfare. There was no moment where a bell rang or a banner dropped from the ceiling saying, "Congratulations, you've just survived cancer." Normalcy just . . . shifted. Again. Gradually. Almost invisibly.

At first, Wendi stayed horizontal. Sleep was her default setting. She drifted in and out with the rhythm of someone caught between exhaustion and refusal to stop progressing. I learned to listen to her breaths, not for problems but for patterns: when they were shallow, when they deepened, when they paused mid-sentence.

Then came the first signs.

She asked for water before I offered. She sat up without needing support. One morning, she walked—slowly, unsteadily—into the kitchen to make some green tea. That moment should have felt mundane. It didn't. It felt like a small resurrection.

Her physical recovery was stunning. Day by day, she reclaimed mobility. Strength. Color. She still moved like someone carrying invisible bruises, but the weight of illness was less visible now. She was in pain but eager to press into more freedom with each passing day. Her hair began to regrow—not in long waves but in short, stubborn defiance. It initially came back to her in a very curly fashion. While she continued to wear a wig in social settings, she rarely wore one at home. Around family, she let the fuzz sit atop her head like a badge.

But it was the mental shift that caught me off guard.

She began turning herself into the "yes girl," literally saying yes to anything. And anyone.

An invitation to coffee? Yes. A random midweek dinner with friends? Yes. A group hike? Yes. Golf? Yes—even though she had hated this game precancer and didn't know the difference between a driver and a wedge. Golfing it was. But so much more. She said yes to life with a velocity that made me dizzy. As if time was no longer on our side, and silence was a luxury she could no longer afford.

At first, I thought it was joy. And, I am sure, part of it was. She had, after all, skipped the better part of sixteen months. But beneath the excitement of truly living again lived something deeper. A refusal.

She was refusing to go back to who she was before cancer. The woman who had organized her family's lives, managed everyone's emotions, and rarely let her guard down. The one who so often said no—not because she didn't want to go but because she didn't want to be a burden or leave things undone at home. That woman was nowhere in sight.

Now she said yes because she might not get another chance. And she was going to take full advantage.

Her worry evaporated in ways I couldn't understand. Things that used to annoy her—an untidy counter, an unresolved conversation, a social post not timely read—barely registered with her. She laughed more. She forgave faster. She embraced interruption, spontaneity, and the faces of strangers like they were sacred.

At one point, I watched her laugh—genuinely laugh—at something small and silly with a family member. The sound startled me. It had been so long since I'd heard that type of frequency from her. A sound so innocent. So unguarded.

It wasn't that she'd forgotten the pain. Or the journey. She simply refused to give it control.

But here's the one thing that no one tells you, nor talks about openly: Recovery is not a team sport.

A Rather Big Unveiling

Her newfound and unbridled joy didn't pull me forward. Her constant stream of "yes" didn't feel like freedom to me. It was, instead, creating distance.

I was still hearing the sounds of rigors echoing in my memory. I still smelled hospital bleach when I passed the laundry room. I still studied every facial expression, waiting for signs of pain or discomfort. There was no "off" button. The sentry doesn't automatically deactivate just because the war appears over.

On the outside, it looked like the danger had passed. A bullet dodged. The war was won.

On the inside, at least for me, this was far from reality. For me, unfortunately, a different kind of battle had begun. And, as I had done for so long, I packed this reality in, keeping it hidden and to myself. I didn't want to get in her way. I didn't want to bring her down or step in the way of her being the *yes girl.*

While she was slowly reclaiming the pieces of her body and life, I was realizing how much of myself I had packed away. How many emotions I had crammed down deep into a bunker of my own making. How many visuals I now absolutely refused to revisit. How many memories I had forced myself to forget. All done in the name of protection.

I played the role of sentry, and I played it well. Eyes always forward. Steady and focused. Unshakeable. And now, with the adrenaline gone and the chaos behind us, I was left standing in a quiet house, surrounded by the echo of the wars waged.

Wendi had a clear vision and direction for her new normal. She craved it and moved toward it. She deserved it all. For me, it was so different. I was quietly with her but merely a shell of who I used to be. I felt very alone in my quest to find out what was wrong with me and why I couldn't feel the joy she felt. While she so aggressively stepped forward into yes, I began quietly withdrawing into no.

She was reclaiming this new version of normalcy, holding on to it with both hands and rejoicing in it. It was a bummer that, for now, this version of normalcy was a table for one.

And then it happened.

The yes girl had committed us to a trip to Cabo San Lucas, a weekend with good friends, some golf, a few drinks, and long views of the Sea of Cortez. She seemed relaxed, even with the wig and a baseball cap pulled low. But as the weekend unfolded and her comfort with the crew expanded, something shifted.

On Sunday morning, she walked into the living room without the wig.

I was stunned. Maybe I wasn't ready. But there she was, standing in front of all of us, rubbing her hair. Yes, her hair. The short, stubborn, curly hair that had returned in defiance.

The women leapt up immediately, hugging her, cheering her on. The men stood and reassured her, telling her how good she looked. A few tears flowed: hers, theirs.

And the gent formerly known as the sentry? I simply froze.

Instead of feeling joy in the big moment, I felt myself withdrawing, climbing deeper into the emotional cave I'd carved out for myself. I still can't fully explain it. This moment should have been a celebration, a milestone. Seeing her without a wig in public was supposed to signal a new normal, a forward-leaning step, a resurrection of sorts.

But I wasn't ready. Maybe I was hurt that we hadn't talked about this beforehand. But that sure sounds awfully soft. Or maybe—and this is the part that stings—the deep isolation I had built around myself had become its own comfort zone.

And big moments like this one didn't pull me out. Instead, they served to push me further in.

True Healing

For a few years after her recovery, the yes girl was in full swing. Literally. She continued to pursue golf, and before long, the real athlete in our family was outdriving most men. She wanted to travel, say yes to every invite, be at every event, and try new things. We continued to split our time: fall and winter in Scottsdale, late spring and summer in McCall. From the outside, it looked like we had it all rolling. And we did. At least, she did.

Each annual checkup brought a little more relief, another inch closer to that coveted five-year mark, where remission becomes something real, something earned. And I was there, beside her. For most of it. But yet, I wasn't. I was not present, definitely not in the moment.

Like the old sentry, I could still play a role. But this new role sucked, mostly because I didn't understand it. I was emotionally disconnected, constantly assessing what the hell was wrong with me.

I didn't realize how far I'd fallen until I tried to explain how well I was doing. I smiled at the right times. I used all the right words: grateful, hopeful, tired but good. The fact that I so overused and relied on "good" should have been my first clue. I even cracked a few jokes when people asked how things were. I'd mastered the art of surface living—sounding human without actually being one. She was clearly moving in one direction, up, creating distance between us.

Inside, I was gone. Vanished. Emptied out. And then it got worse.

I hadn't packed my emotions away neatly. I had stuffed them into self-generated boxes and shoved them down into the crawlspace of my memory, boarded up the door, and walked away. They weren't resolved. They were just unreachable. The images, the smells, the sounds—they were too much. The clenched fists. The vastly repeated "so cold." The look in her eyes after she slumped in the car seat and vanished into unconsciousness for thirteen seconds, giving an impression that I had lost her forever. The look of confusion after being lifted off an elevator floor. None of it had been processed.

And now it was leaking.

During my private self-audit, which seemed to go on nonstop, I slowly began to realize my memory was slipping. I couldn't remember normal, everyday things: what I'd eaten, whether I had showered, names, dates. My sentences trailed off or were stopped midstream. I started tasks and abandoned them. I lost hours and, yes, entire days in a fog.

I soon realized I was not merely being forgetful, like leaving keys in a drawer and searching the entire house for the damn things. I was starting to forget that I even had keys. It was like certain parts of the movie were gone. Taped over.

Worse, I stopped caring.

Sports—something that once pulsed so consistently through my bloodstream—became static. I'd watch a game, then realize I hadn't absorbed a single moment of it. Music meant nothing. Books gathered dust, as I rarely could read a page and recall the words. I'd scroll through texts and emails, encouraging myself to reply later, something I rarely did.

I stopped initiating plans. Stopped reaching out. Friends gave me space at first, assuming I was decompressing. But I wasn't decompressing. I was detaching.

I kept it to myself. This is what I had done most of my life and, most particularly and aggressively, during my time as a sentry. Even though I was losing it, I remained diligent in protecting the yes girl.

She deserved her return to this new normal. And I wasn't going to stand in the way of this progress.

I conjured up the unthinkable: early-onset dementia? But Jesus, that would be early. I started wondering about physical causes, which launched me even further into the only coping mechanism I had ever leaned on as a crutch—movement. I dove deeper into the gym. Yoga. F45. Peloton. If it had a sweat factor, I was in. I thought maybe I could outrun it. Maybe I could sweat out the fog in my brain. Maybe constant motion would lead to clarity.

Nope.

Being a sentry isn't a temporary role. It rewires you. When your entire identity becomes protecting someone else, there's no road map for who you are once you are no longer needed. When the adrenaline finally drains to empty and you step out of fight-or-flight, it doesn't leave peace. It leaves a vacuum.

Some nights I sat alone on a dark patio, reflecting on how I had arrived at this place. It certainly was not a destination I had chosen, nor one I was prepared to navigate out of.

I did not view myself as suicidal. I wasn't spiraling outward. I was just . . . vacant. Like someone had turned the volume down on life, and I hadn't noticed until I realized I'd stopped dancing.

And because Wendi was thriving, really living and in the moment, I felt ashamed of my retreat. I was still her protector, and I didn't want to ruin her momentum. I certainly did not want to weigh her down. So I faked it. I clapped from the cheap seats of her new life, cheering her return while quietly folding further into my own personal absence.

Sensing something was up, a close friend, and the *yes girl* herself, pushed me into something I never would've chosen: a hike at the Grand Canyon. The hike part? That fit nicely. That was my current speed. Constant movement. But the rest of the trip? A weekend in an RV? Now that was a bit outside my wheelhouse. Turns out, the RV part was pretty damn cool.

The hike was stunning, complete with good company, crisp spring air, and one of the greatest wonders of the world spread out before me in all its glory. But somewhere between the rim and the river, I felt more lost than ever. Disoriented. Alone. Even amid the beauty of it all, I felt off. Not myself.

I still wouldn't say I was suicidal, but I definitely found myself in a close neighborhood. A few blocks over. But perhaps in the same zip code. It was while completing the long climb up, body aching and mind continuing to unravel, that I made a decision: It was time to seek help.

P.T.S. What?

First, I started in familiar territory: a medical doctor. Off I went to my general practitioner's office for an annual physical. As with most of these visits, I started in the waiting area, mindlessly filling out forms. I did notice this one seemed different, but it didn't change my approach of mindlessly answering prompted questions. Maybe it was a post-COVID thing, but this form included a short mental health questionnaire—ten or so questions asking how I was feeling in different ways. Most were asking me to rate my feelings on a scale, and I went about the answers truthfully but not thoughtfully.

After my physical exam and an "All looks good" comment, my doctor asked me to join him in his office. This did not feel unusual, and we started off talking about mountain biking. Then he asked, almost casually, if I'd ever used what I called "happy pills," my name for prescriptive anxiety and depression pills. I told him no. He could tell I was growing more anxious. He came out and suggested that I consider such a pill and assured me I could start with a "child-sized dose." While he wasn't pushing hard on this, he also wasn't backing off.

Eventually, he made his way to the questionnaire. "You scored low," he said.

"How low?" I asked.

"Deep depression low," he came back without any hesitation. Damn. Didn't see that coming. After a bit more dialogue, I left with a prescription for some happy pills and a pill cutter to make my own child-sized dose. Given I was also a bit shocked by my score on the depression meter, I also left with a quiet resolve to push my help envelope a bit further.

I was going to talk to a psychologist. My first such trip.

Since we were about to jump on happy pills, why not try out some couch time? Up until then, my "therapist" had been the bar stool next to a close friend. Or the gym. Or running a marathon. Or scripture. But an actual therapist? This was foreign territory for me.

A quick Google search landed me a name, and I got very lucky. That name turned out to be exactly a match. Apprehensive but willing, I showed up. That alone was a big step. I walked in with a small chip on my shoulder, which showed in my opting for a chair rather than the couch. And I didn't say much at first. It took until session two (of five) to crack open the safe and, therefore, my protective layer. By session three, maybe a few tears appeared. Maybe. By session four, a diagnosis, and following session five, options for a plan.

That was it. Five sessions. A diagnosis and options for a plan. Sounds simple, eh? Nothing ever is.

The verdict? Dissociative amnesia, a form of PTSD.

It is a condition often linked to trauma survivors, especially those who aren't the patient but the protector. A sentry, perhaps? Caregivers. The ones who hold everything together when someone else is falling apart. As caregivers, we absorb everything. Then we forget. Not because we want to but because our brains don't give us a choice.

At first, it didn't make sense. But as she described it further, the cause caught my attention, and it could not have hit any closer to home. Here is my version of this form of PTSD, in plain English, likely missing all kinds of clinical nuance. But this worked for me.

If you live in fight-or-flight for a prolonged period, that's no bueno. Stay there too long, and things start to break down. If, during that time, you're exposed to moments you never wanted to see, and definitely would never want to revisit, your mind does its job. It protects you by burying the memory. And the shovel. But in the process, it goes too far, and its efforts to shield the tragic events from your memory unintentionally wipe out other memories.

You don't get to hand-select which memories get packed away. You can't trick the mind into erasing the bad and keeping the good. Baby, meet bathwater. The good news? I wasn't experiencing early-onset dementia. The bad news? Memories, both good and bad, were deeply crammed away, causing me confusion in my daily interactions. I was a mess.

In playing the role of sentry, calm on the outside, vigilant inside, I packed away emotions, images, and memories that could stand in the way of protecting my wife. And in doing so, I lost more than just the trauma I so didn't want to revisit. I lost real memories. Important ones. And, for the life of me, I couldn't figure out where they had gone.

That is the cost of the dissociation. I was present in my daily life, but I wasn't in the moment. I could play the part, smile at the right times, nod along, but deep down I was lost in the gaps. Confused. Trying desperately to sort out why the good memories felt out of reach too.

Studies show that when trauma is sustained over weeks, months, or years, the brain's memory systems begin to malfunction. Certain regions of the brain (like the hippocampus and prefrontal cortex) stop playing nicely together. Memories don't vanish. They just . . . bury themselves. Think of it like a file you saved somewhere, but the folder disappeared.

The idea of dissociative amnesia made little sense until I understood the cause. Then it became a bullseye.

It wasn't like one day, I woke up screaming or forgetting my own name. I just slowly stopped remembering how I felt during those long months in battle. I could recall the logistics—the treatments, medications, rigors—but not the feeling of being there. Sort of like watching footage of your own life with the sound turned off.

Caregivers—especially men—aren't often told that this is a thing. We encourage ourselves to "man up," "power through," and take pride in our stoicism. We tend to see our silence and unwillingness to share as a strength. But silence becomes isolation. And isolation eventually collapses.

You can only carry someone else's survival for so long before your own footing gives way. You often hear it takes a village. Maybe I should have let more of my village in.

For any trained psychologist reading this, I'm sure I am oversimplifying. Maybe I am missing big pieces. This was all new, and just like with the happy pills, I needed to start with a child-sized dose. This was enough and, frankly, all I could handle. Enough to start understanding. Enough to begin the process of coming back to myself.

Process of Unpacking

After leaving my psychologist for the fifth and final session—my decision, not her recommendation—I walked out holding on to three potential paths to start the healing process. Each one was a way to begin unpacking. To start cleaning out the basement in my mind and soul, where so many memories, good and bad, were packed away like old boxes no one wanted to open. Not just memories but a boatload of emotions. I was in for a spring cleaning on steroids.

Bring on the happy pills.

I started taking my child-sized dose of happy pills daily, then threw myself into projects. My wife seemed pleased with this. Not with the pills but with the projects. First came the new deck on our patio. More happy pills. Same dose. Then I painted the inside of a three-car garage—by hand, with a roller and a pole. More happy pills, with some Advil tossed in for good measure. We had talked about adding flagstone steps leading to a flagstone patio in the yard for a firepit. Why not? More happy pills. A lot more Advil.

There was a method to this madness. The work, most performed solo, cleared my mind. It gave me space to think, to start reckoning with how I had gotten here and how the role of sentry brought me to this point. Compromised. Wounded. But finally ready to heal. *Really* heal.

During that fifth and final session, my therapist had outlined three options to help me address dissociative amnesia:

1. Psychedelic mushrooms (I know there are lots of names for this, but I am just calling a spade a spade);

2. Eye movement desensitization and reprocessing (EMDR), or "eye/light therapy."

3. A deep, conscious effort to unpack the trauma manually.

On the surface, all sounded awful. Each one required stepping outside my comfort zone, something I didn't exactly enjoy. But I tried to keep an open mind and carefully worked through the list while I lined up the intense chores I took on that summer.

Option one was eventually eliminated. I am a control freak when it comes to my body, and psychedelics can absolutely mess with control. This is likely what they are designed to do. Losing grip, even temporarily, was too much of a leap. This became a hard pass.

Option two was intriguing but . . . confusing. Eye movement triggered by light patterns was supposed to help unlock memory? Even if it worked, it didn't make any sense to me. While the thought of letting light do the real work was intriguing, if I couldn't understand the mechanism, I couldn't buy in. I eliminated option two.

This left me with an answer and left Wendi with some serious home improvements. I landed on option three, knowing full well that this spring cleaning was not going to be easy. This was going to require me to roll up my sleeves. It sounded like a ton of work, like cleaning out a cluttered attic. I knew I would run into things I didn't want to see. But I also knew how good it could feel when the job was done. That feeling when the shelves are clean, the boxes are labeled, and the space feels open and light again. By the end of the summer, I was ready to do the work.

It was time for some spring cleaning of the mind and soul.

After leaving McCall that summer, chores done and Advil bottles empty, I landed back in Scottsdale, ready to go to work on myself. But how? How do you unpack a mind and soul that's been jam-packed for years? I considered various self-help books, podcasts, and other forms of structured help. I even considered a return visit to my therapist. But the control freak in me would not permit this. I needed to be the one behind the wheel, deciding how far and how fast this thing would go.

Late summer turned into fall. Fall crept into winter. Holidays. All good reasons to delay.

I started the process by making one decision. I decided to jump off the happy pills. My doctor had told me that, if I reached that decision, I needed to work with him to develop a strategy to wean myself off. Going cold turkey could create complications. However, when I called him, he laughed. "Off of what?" he joked. Cutting a child's dose into four pieces would likely require a liquid dropper. Happy pills were done.

All the while, during my delay and avoidance, I continued to do what I'd learn to do so well. I kept playing the role. I'd done it so well as a sentry, so why not keep going? Why not fake my way through the small, intimate interactions that came with daily life? It was becoming second nature. But down deep, I knew the answer. Fake it until you make it only delays the inevitable. I had real work to do.

Unpacking it all wasn't a cinematic moment. There was no big realization, no teary catharsis. I didn't hear trumpets in the distance. Just small cracks. Little ruptures in the dam I had built. An image I could no longer unsee. A story I'd tell and suddenly know how it ends.

These little steps led me back to a place I felt most comfortable. With myself. In a quiet room. With a leather journal my Mama Bear daughter had purchased for me that Christmas. Not knowing what I wanted to write about at first, I started with our normalcy prior to the gut punch. Then I wrote about the diagnosis and the challenge of Face-Timing the kids. I started picking up steam and energy with every page, going old-school with pen and paper. The more I wrote, the more I recalled. The more I recalled, the more I remembered. Whether painful or not, memories and emotions were slowly being pulled from the depths of my mind. Page by page, morning after morning, these memories hit paper, and a bit more of myself was reclaimed.

It was with a pace and energy not seen in years that I attacked that journal, filling pages without looking back, most of the time leaving me unsure as to what I had written. But write I did, feeling more joyful of the time we had in front of us. Strength slowly returned, followed by a weak but present form of confidence. After that, I *wanted* to resurface, but only when the pen was down for the day.

I became passionate about my writing, not only for healing but for the renewed sense of purpose it offered me. I was viewing myself as something other than a caregiver. And, slowly, my words pulled pieces of me back. Not all at once. Not cleanly. But enough to recognize myself again. Each memory I faced was like a hand reaching into the fog, pulling me home. Each sentence was a breadcrumb.

For me, true healing didn't begin the day she got better. I see that now. It began the day I stopped pretending I had.

The zeal and commitment I showed in my writing sparked an internal blaze, leading me from the journal to my phone, then to my laptop. And when the pen finally rested, my motivation was to share this journey, if only to attempt to create a willingness to discuss the aftereffects a caregiver may have. And this process made me want to aggressively avoid further avoidance.

But before I did, I had more learning to do. More avoidance to attack. After all, there are stages: crawl, walk, run. I was far from running. Remember the condo we owned in Boise, the one attached to the infamous elevator where she passed out? I sold it. Avoidance. The McCall home, where I vividly remember her staring at the ceiling fan? Sold. Avoidance.

And now, we were back in Scottsdale, ground zero. Living in the home where so many battles had been fought. What was to become of that place? The place I slept on the couch, avoided the bedroom, and still saw strands of clipped hair on our back patio?

You guessed it. I contacted a realtor.

And Mayo? Easy. I avoided driving anywhere near it. And when I couldn't avoid the route, I merely refused to look in that direction, acting as though it didn't exist. Avoidance. That was the game I played with myself. But as I took stock of how tightly I was clinging to those patterns, I realized one crucial thing: Maybe this is where I needed to begin my cleaning.

So I contacted our realtor and let her know I decided to stay put. After that, slowly, I spent more time in the bedroom. I reminded myself that it was just a room. Not the cause.

Then came the first night I would spend in that room. Then the second. And the third.

Next, I didn't just drive in the direction of Mayo. I drove directly to it. I parked and walked in. I looked around. And then, I decided to drive home, taking the exact path we had taken that day when we were disobeying every traffic rule known to mankind, desperately transporting her limp body to the ER.

This became my chosen method. Head-on. A systematic attack on the avoidance itself. One memory at a time. One room. One route. One trigger. All of it.

It wasn't easy. Avoiding the avoidance meant letting those packed-away emotions resurface. Letting the memories reveal themselves, to be seen again. Letting them take over, even briefly, just long enough to generate reexposure. To reclaim them.

Eventually, this path of head-on included facing the *yes girl* herself. The actress formerly known as the unicorn. The love of my life.

Yes, even with her, I had practiced some level of avoidance. After all, I had been her sentry. Not her husband. Not her lover. Her sentry. Her stoic protector.

The way I now saw her may have been the hardest part to address head-on. Just like the decision to stay in the house, I knew I needed a major reset.

Recognizing that truth was the hard part. But once I did, the change came naturally. After all, love, partnership, and playful intimacy had always been our normal. Since we were twenty-two.

So I started small. Date nights. I let myself hold her again, just a simple hug at first, trusting that I wouldn't break her. Slowly, I began to realize that we could reclaim what we had before the gut punch.

And that slow, deliberate process of seeing her not as a patient, not as someone I needed to protect, but as my wife, proved to be the most meaningful step I could take toward healing.

Every day became a step in that transformation. And with every difficult memory that came flooding back, a good one typically accompanied it. I'd always believed you have to take the good with the bad. Now, more than ever, I was living that belief. And as I gained experience and regained my footing, I could accept this. After all, those good ones could be cherished again.

The Last Sweep

No one picks their ultimate path. Instead, the path is determined by unanticipated circumstances. While you don't select your path, you do control how you manage the walk.

Still unsure how we landed here, so far from our previous normal, we both began picking up the pieces, albeit not always together. Like it or not, this was our newly introduced normal. And within this new normal, it was time to decide who we were now.

The house was quiet in a way that made everything else louder. Footsteps echoed. Drawers closed with finality. Appliances seemed to hum more noticeably. Wendi moved through rooms with a quiet purpose, gathering chargers, organizing drawers, removing bits of fabric from the couch, as if reclaiming small parts of herself that had been left behind in the blur.

I followed behind, slower. Not physically, but emotionally. I found myself watching her every movement. Taking in the quiet. And I kept thinking, *How did we land here?*

We survived the same storm—her storm—but washed ashore in very different places. I now envied her clarity of purpose, even as I understood it had cost her plenty to get there. After weathering such a deep recalibration of our lives, it was inevitable we'd see ourselves—and each other—through changed eyes.

Spending time together in our Scottsdale home now felt like the closing scene of a film neither of us remembered auditioning for. It had started in panic, unfolded in desperate battles, and ended with both a celebration and deep exhaustion. Gratitude was embraced by both of us, given the odds she overcame. But there was something quieter that we felt yet never discussed. There was an awareness that we were walking into slightly different versions of the future.

And maybe that was okay.

What no one tells you is that survival doesn't guarantee symmetry. You can overcome the gut punch, pull so closely together to navigate the treatment journey, only to wind up in different places on the other side. You can both live past the journey and come away changed in ways that don't align.

We were still us. Still tethered. Thirty-five years and counting. Still deeply connected. But something had shifted—subtly, likely permanently.

Her eyes now saw opportunities. Mine still scanned for threats. I was looking for storm clouds on the horizon, but she was seeing postcard days ahead. She looked ahead. I kept glancing back, not out of regret but instinct. I was still unlearning the reflex to guard, watch, prepare.

And the truth is, our paths may never fully align again.

Coming to that realization didn't bring sadness. It brought relief. Because, after the journey, maybe alignment isn't the goal.

Maybe, after life stalls and shifts so suddenly, the goal is motion. Forward. Not in lockstep, not in symmetry, but in mutual movement. As long as neither of us is stuck—knee-deep in mud or silence—we can push forward, together. Movement is the new normal, provided both of us can be mentally present. We don't have to walk the same road at the same speed.

We just need to keep walking.

Converging Paths Ahead

I'm not sure alignment ever truly arrives. The yes girl got a head start on reclaiming her new normal, while I was still tucked away in my isolation cave. But as I emerged, I began to notice something unexpected: At times, our paths did converge. And in those moments, I relearned how to be in the moment—with her, with loved ones, and with my own experiences.

And if I have one more dirty little secret to share, this one is actually a remarkable one.

After picking up the broom and sweeping out the deeply stored memories and emotions, the next appropriate step is true emergence from the isolation cave. And when that step is taken—when you allow yourself to be present again—something surprising awaits.

The colors seem more vibrant. Jokes seem funnier. Stories seem more interesting. The world seems more . . . alive.

It's a rainbow after a storm. A prize at the bottom of a cereal box. A simple, powerful reminder that presence itself may be the reward for surviving what you never expected to face.

Your ability to be present—fully, genuinely present—is what awaits after your emergence from isolation.

And that is a good secret worth sharing.

A Former Sentry's Final Take

We didn't say much as we got into the car. We rarely did now. Nearly two years had passed since the end of her aggressive treatment plan—enough time for her body to heal but not enough for either of us to fully make sense of the toll it had taken. The silence between us wasn't emptiness; it was residue, what remained after the battle was waged. And now, it was time to relocate again for the summer months.

The doors closed with that familiar, weighted click. I glanced over at her, hair restored, makeup back in the game, clothing now selected for fashion, not necessity. She stared out the window, quiet, eyes fixated on something distant. Maybe the lake. Maybe a thought she hadn't spoken yet. Maybe a "yes" she was looking forward to.

As I pulled out of the driveway, I looked back at our Scottsdale home, seeing it now as a home and not a battlefield. That, in and of itself, was a major milestone.

A sports talk show played on the radio, neither of us listening or paying any attention. Sounds like this were merely to fill gaps. After all, as we continued walking down slightly different paths, conversations had more gaps, something we were growing accustomed to.

She turned to me, just for a second, and smiled—not the full kind, not the one that showed teeth. Just a soft smile. A real smile. No mask.

I smiled back, something that was coming easier these days. No words were exchanged.

And this was enough.

Other than heading back toward McCall, neither one of us truly knew where we were going—not emotionally, not spiritually. How could we? But we were moving.

And for now, that was also enough.

For what it is worth, here's my reclaimed self's take: Adversity breeds growth. With growth comes the opportunity for greater achievement. Sure, I sometimes mourn the normal we had. But the adversity we both endured brought something else too. It forced growth. And that growth cracked open doors we didn't even know existed. Like Wendi crushing a golf ball 250 yards down a fairway. Like me writing a memoir. Real growth previously not imagined.

Maybe this evolving version of "normal," shaped by survival and resilience, comes with a higher ceiling. A higher ceiling for joy. For presence in each moment. For connection. Maybe that's the trade. If so, bring on the gut punch, in whatever form it takes.

For me, the biggest transformation came in learning to stop avoiding. That was my growth. A close friend helped me get there. He encouraged me to start every day by eating the frog. Translation: Do the thing you're most tempted to avoid. It was life-changing for me.

The journey is painful. But the growth? Exponential. It led to greater emotional depth, greater love, and, yes, even greater joy.

And one more thing . . . fuck cancer.

JUST HOW FAST NORMAL CAN DRAMATICALLY CHANGE

Talk about zero to sixty, with respect to a collapsing normal. This is the speed we shifted from entering a much-needed, post-COVID spring to abruptly moving into our new normal as caregiver and cancer patient.

January 27, 2021: First call to healthcare provider expressing concern regarding a lump.

February 8, 2021: Appointment for mammogram.

March 2, 2021: Follow-up appointment for ultrasound and additional imaging.

March 5, 2021: First gut punch, informed that Wendi had breast cancer.

March 8, 2021: Second gut punch, doctor using term "triple-negative breast cancer."

March 17, 2021: First meetings with the medical team at Mayo Clinic.

March 22, 2021: First walk into the infusion room for chemotherapy.

FOR THE NEXT SENTRY

Things I Wish I Knew When Treatment Began

When the storm first hits, everyone looks to you, the sentry. You'll be told to stay strong, to be her anchor. And you'll do that, because you must. But here are some things I wish someone had told me before I stepped into the fight.

You can't prepare for the storm, but you can fortify your post. Build your network early: medical, emotional, practical. You'll need people who can stand in for you when you can't see straight, who remind you to eat, who notice when you're unraveling. Isolation is part of the new normal, but widen the net a bit. That's not weakness. It's readiness.

You're not being strong by staying silent. Holding everything in may feel like control, but it's a quiet form of collapse. Find at least one person you can talk to without editing yourself. Call them your guardian angel. They will cherish the term and the role. Even sentries need to unburden themselves.

Write things down. Appointments, medications, reactions—yes, document the shit out of those. But also record the moments you think you'll never forget. Because you will. And one day, when the fog lifts, you'll be grateful for a written map of where you've been.

Ask every question twice. You'll only hear half the answer the first time. Fear, fatigue, and hope all distort clarity. Ask again. Doctors are used to it. You are not being difficult. You're being thorough.

Don't let the system rush your humanity. Speed matters, but presence matters too. Take five minutes before each decision to breathe, to look at her, to remind yourself why you're there. And how you got there. This isn't just a medical journey. It's a human one as well.

Rigors, reactions, and side effects aren't just clinical events. They're trauma in motion—for her and for you. Bear witness. Describe what you see. If only to yourself. It helps doctors and nurses, but it also helps you process what the mind will later so desperately try to bury.

You'll be asked, "How's she doing?" far more often than, "How are you holding up?" Answer both. Even if the second answer is quiet and rushed, whisper the answer to yourself later. Out loud. This becomes an early and very necessary form of unpacking, while still in the middle of the fight.

Accept help before you think you need it. You will need it. Without any doubt. If you are not ready to seek outside help, start small. Let others run errands, cook meals, sit with her while you walk outside and breathe some air that doesn't smell like antiseptic. You can't stand guard forever without some rest.

You're deep in fight-or-flight. Make no big decisions outside of the fight. The person making choices now is a version of you built for survival. You are a stoic sentry. He's sharp, laser-focused, protective, but he's also exhausted and reactive. Protect your future self from making decisions you will regret later while you are in this dense fog.

One day, the battle will go quiet, and that silence will test you. When the treatments end and the noise fades, you'll expect relief. Instead, you may find disorientation. You've spent months living by alarms and lab results; when those stop, you may not know who you are. That's not weakness. That's the body and mind finally trying their best to play catch-up. Don't isolate further. That is where the real danger is waiting.

You never asked for this role. No one ever does.

But here you are: standing guard beside someone you love while the world as you knew it dissolves around you. You will move through each day with an urgency that feels unnatural, fueled by instinct, duty, and a fear you'll try hard not to name. You will learn to read the room, lab numbers, expressions, and silences. You will learn to wait.

You will discover how quickly the mind adapts—how things that once seemed unbearable become routine. You'll speak a new language of side effects and scan results, while the rest of the world goes on discussing weather, work, and plans for the weekend. The distance between those worlds will widen until you barely recognize the one you lived in previously.

There will be days when you hold your breath for hours at a time, afraid to exhale in case something changes while you do. You'll become fluent in vigilance, hyperaware of every sound coming from the next room. And yet, despite your focus, you'll miss things—small things, emotional things—because survival mode makes it impossible to feel everything at once.

Don't mistake that numbness for weakness. It's what the body and mind do to keep you upright.

When the storm finally breaks—and it will—you may think the hardest part is behind you. But the quiet that follows brings its own weight. The silence will ask questions you don't yet have the strength to answer. You'll try to return to your old life, but the colors and pace feel different. The world has changed while you were a sentry. You feel lost. And, surprise, the world is not the only thing that has changed. You've changed too.

And when the time comes where you can finally rest—*really* rest—give yourself permission to unravel. The body can only stay armored for so long. Healing, for both of you, will come at different paces. And true healing will take time and grace.

You'll need to find strength for the long, quiet work of finding your way back home. Not to your previous normal; that world is long gone. But instead, to a shifted normal, where your adversity becomes a tool for growth, for expansion. To love more deeply and appreciate more fully.

www.ingramcontent.com/pod-product-compliance
Lightning Source LLC
LaVergne TN
LVHW090412210926
848480LV00002B/536
* 9 7 9 8 8 9 7 4 7 0 6 5 5 *